Radiographic Atlas of Cardiac Implantable Electronic Devices

Radiographic Atlas of Cardiac Implantable Electronic Devices

Majid Haghjoo, MD

Professor, Cardiac Electrophysiologist, Department of Cardiac Pacing and Electrophysiology, Rajaie Cardiovascular Medical and Research Center, Tehran, Iran

Farzad Kamali, MD

University Faculty and Cardiac Electrophysiologist, Department of Cardiac Pacing and Electrophysiology, Rajaie Cardiovascular Medical and Research Center, Tehran, Iran

Amir Farjam Fazelifar, MD

University Faculty and Cardiac Electrophysiologist, Department of Cardiac Pacing and Electrophysiology, Rajaie Cardiovascular Medical & Research Center, Tehran, Iran

ELSEVIER

Elsevier
1600 John F. Kennedy Blvd.
Ste 1800
Philadelphia, PA 19103-2899

Radiographic Atlas of Cardiac Implantable Electronic Devices, First edition   ISBN: 978-0-323-84753-7

Notices

Practitioners and researchers must always rely on their own experience and knowledge in evaluating and using any information, methods, compounds or experiments described herein. Because of rapid advances in the medical sciences, in particular, independent verification of diagnoses and drug dosages should be made. To the fullest extent of the law, no responsibility is assumed by Elsevier, authors, editors or contributors for any injury and/or damage to persons or property as a matter of products liability, negligence or otherwise, or from any use or operation of any methods, products, instructions, or ideas contained in the material herein.

Content Strategist: Robin R Carter
Editorial Project manager: Tracy I. Tufaga
Project Manager: Kiruthika Govindaraju
Designer: Alan Studholme

 Working together
to grow libraries in
developing countries

www.elsevier.com • www.bookaid.org

Last digit is the print number: 9 8 7 6 5 4 3 2 1

Contents

Biography

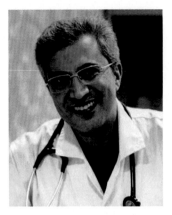

Majid Haghjoo received his fellowship degree in the field of cardiac electrophysiology from Iran University of Medical Sciences with two complementary training courses at the Leipzig Heart Center (Germany) and Ospedale San Raffaele of Milan (Italy) and is currently teaching cardiac electrophysiology at the Rajaie Cardiovascular, Medical and Research Center. His professional interests are focused on atrial fibrillation, ventricular tachycardia, and cardiac resynchronization therapy. In addition, he serves as the director of the Electrophysiology Department at the Rajaie Cardiovascular, Medical and Research Center and is a member of the American College of Cardiology, the European Society of Cardiology, the Heart Rhythm Society, and the European Heart Rhythm Association.

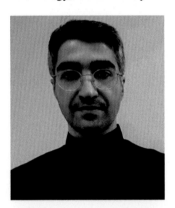

Farzad Kamali received his fellowship degree in the field of cardiac electrophysiology from Iran University of Medical Sciences. He started his career as a cardiac electrophysiologist at the Rajaie Cardiovascular, Medical and Research Center in 2018. He is currently working as an associate professor at this center. His professional interests are in the fields of lead extraction and PVC ablation.

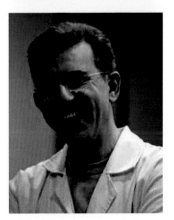

Amir Farjam Fazelifar graduated in the field of cardiac electrophysiology from Iran University of Medical Sciences. He works as an associate professor in a state hospital, Rajaie Cardiovascular, Medical and Research Center. His research and teaching experience is in the fields of cardiac electrophysiology and cardiac electronic device management. He has written a chapter on cardiac electrophysiology in the book *Practical Cardiology*. He is a member of the Iranian Heart Association.

Preface

Several cardiac implantable electronic devices have been developed for use in cardiac rhythm management over the last few decades. Each year more than 1 million cardiac electronic devices are implanted. Chest radiography is a common initial diagnostic method for evaluation of cardiac and pulmonary diseases. Therefore, it is highly likely for cardiologists, cardiac surgeons, internists, pulmonologists, intensivists, pediatricians, and radiologists to encounter a wide variety of these devices on chest radiographs on a daily basis. It is very important for electrophysiologists and electrophysiology fellows and residents to recognize these devices correctly and detect related complications in postimplant and follow-up chest radiographs.

This book is designed to provide a comprehensive atlas of chest radiographs taken from patients with all kinds of currently implanted cardiac electronic devices, including permanent pacemakers, implantable cardioverter defibrillators, cardiac resynchronization therapies (pacemakers and defibrillators), novel devices (subcutaneous defibrillators and wireless pacemakers), and implantable cardiac monitors.

This book also presents a stepwise and user-friendly approach for the diagnostic evaluation of chest radiography in patients with cardiac electronic devices. Briefly, we have attempted to deliver a practical guide to all medical professionals who have an interest in the radiographic presentations of these devices.

It is our hope that readers will find this book to be an essential and valuable tool in the everyday approach to patients with cardiac electronic devices.

Majid Haghjoo, MD, FESC, FACC, FCAPSC
Professor, Cardiovascular Medicine,
Cardiac Electrophysiology Research Center;
Editor-in-Chief, *Research in Cardiovascular Medicine*;
Rajaie Cardiovascular, Medical and Research Center,
Iran University of Medical Sciences, Tehran, Iran

Acknowledgments

This atlas is based on the chest radiographs of patients who had undergone device implantation at our center. I gratefully dedicate this atlas to our patients and our lovely colleagues in the electrophysiology laboratory and radiology departments.

I believe that the completion of this undertaking could not have been possible without the participation and assistance of so many people whose names may not all be enumerated. Their contributions are sincerely appreciated and acknowledged.

On behalf of the coauthors, I thank our families—our wives, Rohangiz, Haleh, and Soma, and our children, Mohammad Amin, Amir Faraz, and Helia—who inspired us with their accompaniment, empathy, sacrifice, and endless love so that we could complete this effort.

Finally, I acknowledge the very committed and compassionate teamwork of Elsevier, especially Robin, Tracy, and Kiruthika who helped us with the first edition of this book.

Majid Haghjoo, MD, FESC, FACC, FCAPSC

General approach for evaluation of cardiac implantable electronic devices

Majid Haghjoo[a,b,*]

[a]*Department of Cardiac Electrophysiology, Rajaie Cardiovascular Medical and Research Center, Iran University of Medical Sciences, Tehran, Iran*
[b]*Cardiac Electrophysiology Research Center, Rajaie Cardiovascular Medical and Research Center, Iran University of Medical Sciences, Tehran, Iran*
Corresponding author: majid.haghjoo@gmail.com

Key Points

- At least two well-penetrated chest radiographic views are necessary for a complete examination of cardiac implantable electronic devices. A posterior–anterior view provides a two-dimensional snapshot of the physical integrity and lead location in the correct chamber. For better evaluation of the lead tip location, a lateral view is also necessary.

- In order to provide a thorough evaluation and complete report, when interpreting chest radiographs containing cardiac implantable electronic devices, physicians should adopt a stepwise approach and make sure all points are addressed.

Introduction

Since the first human implant, several innovative cardiac implantable electronic devices (CIEDs) have been developed [1]. All patients with CIEDs, such as permanent pacemakers (PPMs), implantable cardiac defibrillators (ICDs), cardiac resynchronization therapy (CRT) devices, implantable cardiac monitors (ICMs), leadless pacemakers (LLPs), and novel pacing techniques, undergo chest radiographs (CXRs) on a regular basis. Therefore, it is not uncommon for physicians, residents, and fellows to be presented with a puzzle of CXRs having a variety of these devices in daily practice.

Chest radiography is employed for evaluation of lead location and integrity after CIED implantation as well as for any complications related to their implant [2,3]. At least two well-penetrated CXR views are necessary for a complete examination [4]. A posterior–anterior (PA) view provides a two-dimensional snapshot of the physical integrity and lead location in the correct chamber. For a better evaluation of the lead tip location, a lateral CXR view is necessary. In addition, lateral views allow a distinction to be made between an anteriorly placed right ventricle (RV) lead and a posteriorly coursed left ventricle (LV) lead. It is important to be familiar with conventional PA and lateral CXR cardiac anatomy to distinguish the correct lead locations.

Components of CIED on CXR

A CIED is composed of two main components: a pulse generator encased in titanium and a pacemaker or defibrillator leads. The pulse generator contains the circuitry, a lithium battery, and a connector port (Fig. 1).

The CIED lead has five major parts: a conductor, an insulation (silicone rubber and/or polyurethane), electrode(s), a distal fixation mechanism, and a terminal connector pin. The leads are connected proximally to the generator by the terminal pins through the connecting block. Lead tips may be fixed actively or passively into the myocardium. Leads placed passively have radiolucent "tines" at their ends, which keep the lead tips in position (Fig. 2). With time, the myocardium adjacent to the lead tip undergoes fibrotic change, further stabilizing the lead tip in place.

Active fixation leads have a retractable screw (Fig. 3) at their ends, which is deployed when the connector pin is rotated clockwise by a dedicated torque wrench.

Specific situations in which active fixation is used include RV leads in the interventricular septum (Fig. 4), the outflow tract, or the right-sided ventricle in congenitally corrected transposition of great vessels. In situations, such as free-wall (Fig. 5) or septal implantation or in postcardiac surgery patients, the right atrial (RA) leads must be secured to the tissue for stability.

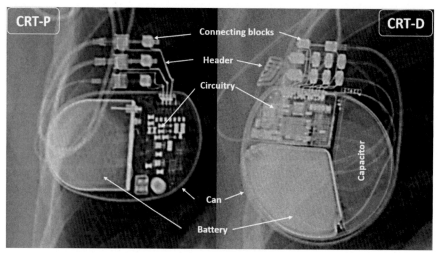

FIG. 1

Basic components of the two cardiovascular implantable electronic device (CIED) generator (one pacemaker and one defibrillator). Generators include a battery, an electronic circuitry, a header containing connector ports, and a capacitor (only in a defibrillator).

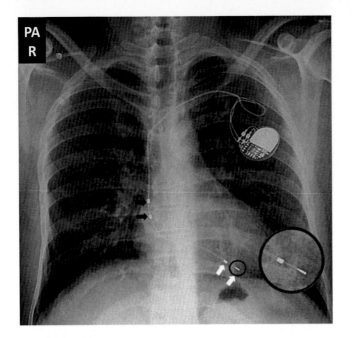

FIG. 2

Passive fixation VDD pacemaker lead. Note that there is no active fixation helix. Passive fixation tines are entirely invisible by X-ray (radiolucent). The distal part of the lead is magnified for better illustration. Floating atrial-sensing electrodes are shown by the *black arrow*, and the sense/pace ventricular electrodes are shown by the *white arrow*.

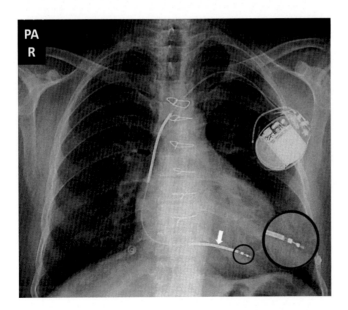

FIG. 3

Active fixation defibrillator lead. Note that the active fixation helix is clearly extended beyond the distal electrode. The distal part of the lead is magnified for better illustration. The superior vena cava coil is shown by the *black arrow*, and the right ventricular electrode is shown by the *white arrow*.

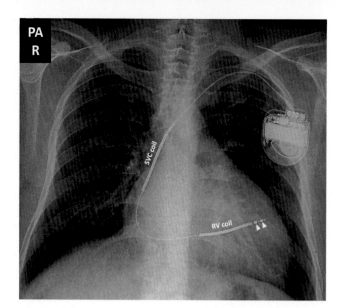

FIG. 4

Septal implantation of the active fixation defibrillator lead in a patient with a single-chamber defibrillator and low R-wave amplitude in the apical area. Note that the defibrillator lead consists of a superior vena cava (SVC) coil, a right ventricular (RV) coil, and sense/pace electrodes (*white arrowheads*).

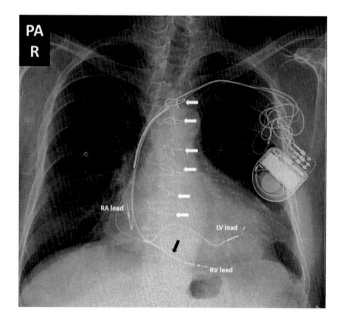

FIG. 5

Free-wall implantation of the active fixation atrial lead in a postcardiac surgery patient with a cardiac resynchronization therapy defibrillator. Note that sternotomy wires are shown by *white arrows*. The active fixation right atrial (RA) lead is implanted in the right atrial free wall and the dual-coil (*black arrows*) right ventricular (RV) defibrillator lead at the RV apex. The left ventricular (LV) passive lead is placed within the free-wall cardiac vein.

Stepwise approach for evaluation of CIED on CXR

In order to assure a thorough evaluation and complete report, when interpreting chest radiographs containing CIEDs, physicians should check the following list and make sure all the points are addressed (Table 1):

Step 1: Determine the device type (pacemaker vs ICD) and the lead numbers: ICDs are easily differentiated from pacemakers by the presence of radiopaque shock coils on the RV leads (Figs. 6–8).

Transvenous ICDs (T-ICDs) are implanted in the pectoral area, and the leads are implanted via a transvenous route and positioned within the cardiac chambers (Fig. 9). However, subcutaneous ICDs (S-ICDs) are implanted in the axillary area,

Table 1 Simplified checklist for CIED evaluation on chest radiographs.

Step	Description
Step 1	Determine the device type (pacemaker versus defibrillator) and the lead numbers
Step 2	Evaluate the terminal connector pin insertion, lead integrity, and positions of the distal electrodes
Step 3	Look for complications (i.e., pneumothorax, hemothorax, lead dislodgement, lead fracture, loose set screw)

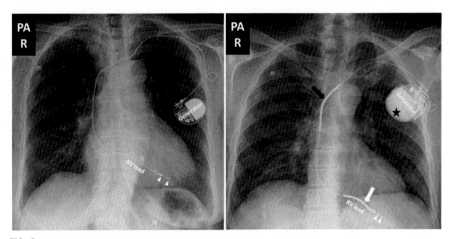

FIG. 6

Comparison between a single-chamber pacemaker and a defibrillator. Note that the pacemaker lead in the right ventricle (RV lead) has only sense/pace electrodes (*white arrowheads*); however, the defibrillator lead (RV lead) has an additional shock coil in the superior vena cava (*black arrow*) and the right ventricular (RV) portions of the lead (*white arrow*). The defibrillator generator is larger than that of the pacemaker and contains a capacitor (*black star*).

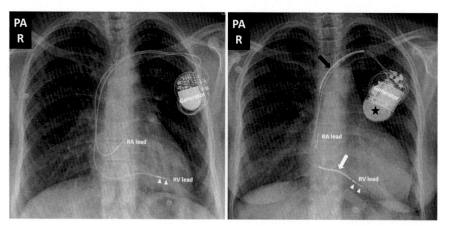

FIG. 7

Comparison between a dual-chamber pacemaker and a defibrillator. Note that the right ventricular (RV) lead in the pacemaker has only sense/pace electrodes (*white arrowheads*); however, the defibrillator lead (RV lead) has an additional shock coil in the superior vena cava (*black arrow*) and the right ventricular (RV) portions of the lead (*white arrow*). The right atrial (RA) leads are similar in the pacemaker and the defibrillator. The defibrillator generator is larger than that of the pacemaker and contains a capacitor (*black star*).

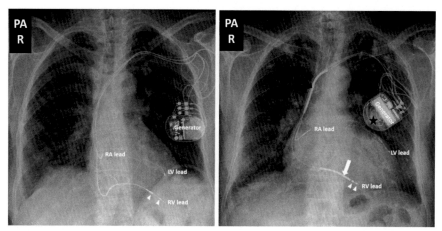

FIG. 8

Comparison between a cardiac resynchronization therapy pacemaker (CRT–P) and a defibrillator (CRT–D). Note that the right ventricular (RV) lead in the CRT-P has only sense/pace electrodes (*white arrowheads*); however, the defibrillator lead (RV lead) has an additional shock coil in the superior vena cava (*black arrow*) and the right ventricular (RV) portions of the lead (*white arrow*). The right atrial (RA) and left ventricular (LV) leads are similar in CRT-P and CRT-D devices. The CRT-D generator contains a capacitor (*black star*).

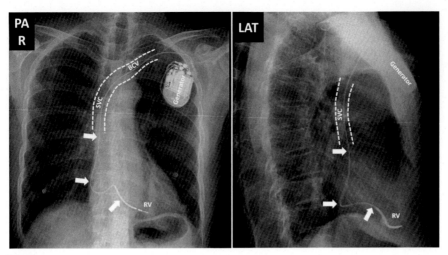

FIG. 9

Posteroanterior (PA) and lateral (LAT) chest radiographic views of a transvenous single-chamber defibrillator. Note that the defibrillator lead (*white arrow*) is implanted transvenously via the brachiocephalic vein (BCV) and the superior vena cava (SVC) within the right ventricular (RV) chamber.

and the leads are implanted subcutaneously in an L-shaped pattern in the left lower chest and in the left parasternal region (Fig. 10). LLPs are completely implanted within the RV cavity and have no separate leads (Fig. 11).

After determining the device type, it is recommended to determine the lead numbers for further classification of CIEDs into single-, dual-, and triple-chamber devices. In this stage, it is very important to confirm lead connection into the generators. Nonfunctional CIED leads are being abandoned in place when they cannot be safely removed. Sometimes several abandoned leads are seen in the CXR of a single patient (Fig. 12). Only connected leads are used to determine the device type.

Step 2: Evaluate the terminal connector pin insertion, lead integrity, and positions of the distal electrodes: to ensure proper CIED system functioning, a careful scrutiny of the CIED leads from terminal pin insertion into the generator to the distal tip is recommended. The proximal end of an electrode has an insertion port that attaches the lead or leads to the generator. The electrode should slightly extend beyond the connecting blocks for the device to function properly (Fig. 13). If it does not, then the electrode must be reconnected.

To reduce the device size, the terminal connector pins in ICD (DF-1 connection) and pacemaker leads (IS-1 connection) are at least partially replaced by the new standard IS-4/DF-4 in new devices (Fig. 14). The DF-1 lead consists of bifurcated (in a single-coil lead) or trifurcated (in a dual-coil lead) terminal connector pins, including a one pace/sense IS-1 connector and one or two DF-1 high-voltage connectors. These connectors join together into a yoke, which then integrates these into a single

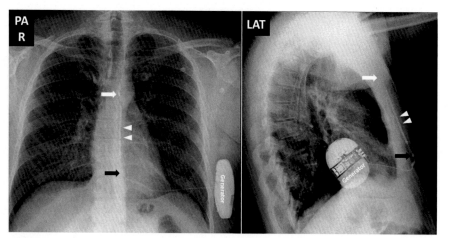

FIG. 10

Posteroanterior (PA) and lateral (LAT) chest radiographic views of a subcutaneous implantable cardioverter defibrillator. Note that the defibrillator lead is implanted subcutaneously in an "L"-shaped pattern in the left parasternal area. The lead has proximal-sensing (*black arrow*) and distal-sensing (*white arrow*) electrodes and one intervening coil (*white arrowhead*).

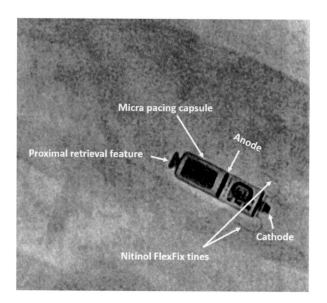

FIG. 11

Micra transcatheter pacing system. Components of a Micra pacing capsule include a cathode, an anode, Nitinol FlexFix tines, and proximal retrieval features.

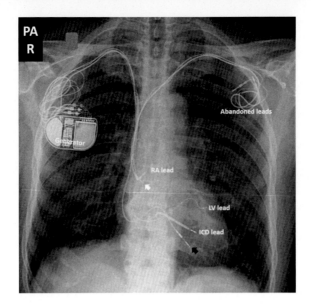

FIG. 12

Abandoned pacing leads. A posteroanterior (PA) chest radiographic view in a patient with a cardiac resynchronization therapy defibrillator (CRT–D) implanted from the right side. Note that the patient had a dual-chamber pacemaker implanted from the left side (the right ventricular lead is shown by the *black arrow*, and the atrial lead is shown by the *white arrow*). During upgrade, the left-sided axillary and subclavian venous system was found to be occluded and the patient did not consent for lead extraction. Therefore, left-sided leads were abandoned in the pocket and a complete CRT-D system was implanted from the right side.

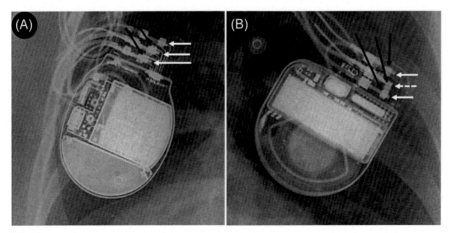

FIG. 13

Close-up view of leads correctly connected into a cardiac resynchronization device (A) and a case of loose connection (B). Connecting blocks are shown by *black arrows*, and terminal pins are shown by a white arrow. Note that all pins in Panel A are clearly extended beyond the connecting blocks; however, the middle pin in Panel B (shown in a *square dot*) is not extended beyond its connecting block.

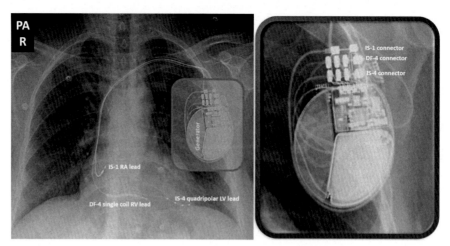

FIG. 14

Close-up view of a connecting block in a cardiac resynchronization therapy defibrillator device. Note that the right atrial (RA) lead is connected through the IS-1 connector, the right ventricular (RV) defibrillator lead through the DF-4 connector, and the left ventricular (LV) through the IS-4 connector.

lead body. The DF-4 lead has only one connector pin with four inline poles (two low-voltage poles for pace/sense and two high-voltage poles for defibrillation coils) and no yoke. Similarly, the IS-4 lead consists of one connector pin with four inline poles (four low-voltage poles for pace/sense) with no yoke.

Normally, the lead should follow a smooth pathway without forming any loops, as it may cause cardiac arrhythmia and even migration and lead dislodgement. In patients with normal anatomic variants such as a persistent left superior vena cava (Fig. 15), the leads may show an abnormal course.

The most common sites for lead fracture are at the lead fixation to the pocket or at the entry of the subclavian vein, where it gets crushed between the clavicle and the first rib (also known as the subclavian crush syndrome). The right atrial (RA) lead should be in the RA appendage. On a PA view, the RA lead has a slight medial course, while on a lateral CXR view, its location is anterior and forms a "J" loop (Fig. 16).

The RV lead on a PA view has its tip pointing toward the cardiac apex or the interventricular septum and should be to the left of the spine, while on the lateral view, the lead should curve along the course of the right atrial lateral wall, passing the tricuspid valve, and pointing anteriorly and slightly inferiorly or superiorly depending on RV apical or septal fixation (Fig. 16).

In patients with CRT devices, it is difficult to differentiate an RV electrode from an LV electrode on a PA view. For this purpose, a lateral CXR view can be more useful. In this case, the RV electrode is located anteriorly, while the LV lead is located at the posterior part of the cardiac silhouette (Fig. 17).

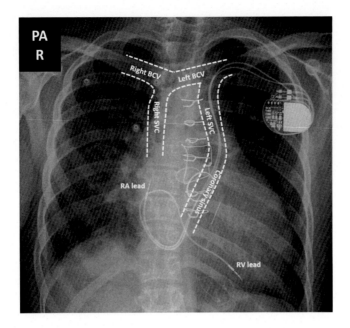

FIG. 15

Posteroanterior (PA) chest radiographic view of a dual-chamber pacemaker in a patient with a persistent left superior vena cava (SVC). Note that the right atrial (RA) and the right ventricular (RV) leads are passed through the left side of the mediastinum via the left SVC rather than via the left brachiocephalic vein (BCV) and the right SVC in the left-sided implant or the right BCV and the right SVC in the right-sided implant.

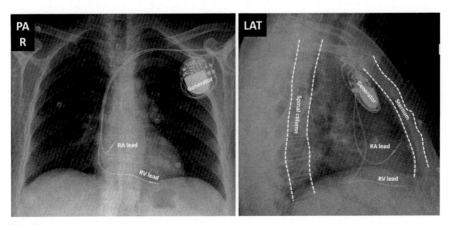

FIG. 16

Posteroanterior (PA) and lateral (LAT) chest radiographic views in a dual-chamber pacemaker. Note that the right atrial (RA) lead has a slight medial course in the PA view; however, its location is anterior and forms a "J" loop in the LAT view. The right ventricular (RV) lead on the PA view has its tip pointing toward the cardiac apex and located to the left of the spine, while on the LAT view, the lead curves along the course of the right atrial lateral wall, passing the tricuspid valve, and pointing anteriorly and slightly inferiorly.

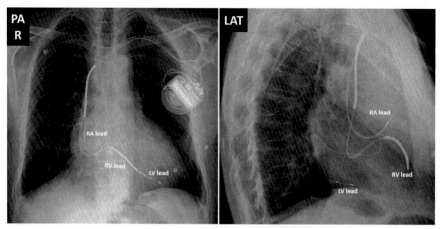

FIG. 17

Posteroanterior (PA) and lateral (LAT) chest radiographic views in a patient with a cardiac resynchronization therapy defibrillator device. Note that the right ventricular (RV) and left ventricular (LV) leads are partially overlapped in the PA view. In the LAT view, the RV electrode is located anteriorly and the LV lead is located in the posterior part of the cardiac silhouette.

Step 3: Look for complications: CIED implantation may be complicated by myocardial perforation, pneumothorax, hemothorax, and lead fracture or dislodgements (please refer to Chapter 5).

References

[1] R. Sutton, J.D. Fisher, C. Linde, D.G. Benditt, History of electrical therapy for the heart, Eur Heart J Suppl 9 (Suppl I) (2007) I3–10.

[2] S.C. Torres-Ayala, G. Santacana-Laffitte, J. Maldonado, Radiography of cardiac conduction devices: a pictorial review of pacemakers and implantable cardioverter defibrillators, J Clin Imaging Sci 4 (2014) 74.

[3] R.P. Mathew, T. Alexander, V. Patel, G. Low, Chest radiographs of cardiac devices (part 1): cardiovascular implantable electronic devices, cardiac valve prostheses and Amplatzer occluder devices, S Afr J Rad 23 (1) (2019), a1730. https://doi.org/10.4102/sajr.v23i1.1730.

[4] A.L. Aguilera, Y.V. Volokhina, K.L. Fisher, Radiography of cardiac conduction devices: a comprehensive review, Radiographics 31 (2011) 1669–1682.

Pacemakers

2

Amir Farjam Fazelifar[a,b,*]

[a]*Department of Cardiac Electrophysiology, Rajaie Cardiovascular Medical and Research Center, Iran University of Medical Sciences, Tehran, Iran*
[b]*Cardiac Electrophysiology Research Center, Rajaie Cardiovascular Medical and Research Center, Iran University of Medical Sciences, Tehran, Iran*
Corresponding author: fazelifar.academic@gmail.com

Key Points

- Every day, different types of pacemakers from several manufacturers are implanted. Chest radiography plays an important role in the correct identification of these devices.
- The main components of pacemakers include a pulse generator and connecting leads.
- Chest radiography helps us to identify the pacemaker type, the lead type, the device manufacturer, the lead course within the heart, and the type of lead fixation to the myocardium.

Introduction

Our story started in 1951, when John Hopps created the first pacemaker. It was an external-portable device and needed to be plugged into power points. Dr. Paul Zoll built an external pacemaker, which was first used in 1952. The first fully implantable pacemaker was built in 1958. In the 1960s and 1970s, a great development occurred in pacemaker technology. Physiologic pacing innovated. It means, chamber pacing, when it is needed (demand pacing) and synchronized atrial and ventricular pacing.

Pacemaker lead design and the technology of pacemaker battery improved in the 1970s. Passive and active fixation in leads and the use of a lithium-iodine battery instead of a mercury oxide-zinc battery were a big success in pacemaker technology [1]. The evolution did not stop there. The next step was creation of rate-responsive pacemakers. A piezoelectric crystal was used to increase the pacing rate during activity.

A new design for leads and delivery system helped to perform left ventricle pacing and biventricular pacing, which showed better cardiac function. This concept was approved clinically in the first years of the 21st century [2].

In 2020, His/LBBB pacing and leadless pacemakers were considered to be top technology. These new technologies have been developing to decrease side effects

Radiographic Atlas of Cardiac Implantable Electronic Devices. https://doi.org/10.1016/B978-0-323-84753-7.00003-0

and to improve outcome after pacemaker implantation. In this chapter, we discuss the radiographic features of different types of pacemaker generators and leads in chest radiography (CXR).

Pacemaker components

A pacemaker has different components, including a generator and leads. Battery, electronics, and connector block are the main parts of a generator (Fig. 1).

Pacemaker leads come in various shapes, length, and type of fixation to the myocardium. On the basis of the manufacturer's logo, shape of the battery, upper and lower borders, header orientation to the battery, and pacemaker connection pins, a Cardiac Rhythm Device Identification Algorithm was developed (Fig. 2) [3].

In clinical practice, the terminal connector block view is highly important. Many pacemaker malfunctions, such as high lead impedance and/or loss of capture, show abnormalities in the terminal connector block.

Pacemaker types

According to the medical indication, we implant pacemakers in different types. Single- or dual-chamber pacemakers can provide sufficient heart rate. Single-chamber pacemakers can be implanted in the right atrium, the right ventricle, or the coronary sinus (Fig. 3).

Dual-chamber pacing is closer to normal physiology. A triple-chamber pacemaker is often used to treat heart failure in certain conditions. In this chapter, we only discuss the radiographic presentations of single- and dual-chamber pacemakers. Triple-chamber pacemakers and leadless pacemakers are covered in Chapters 4 and 6, respectively.

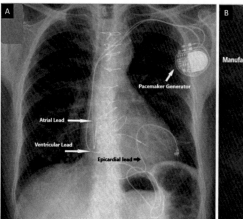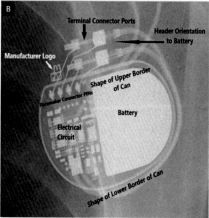

FIG. 1

Panel A: Main components in a dual-chamber pacemaker. *White arrows* show a pacemaker generator and atrial and ventricular leads. The *black arrow* shows an old epicardial lead. Panel B: Details of pacemaker generator structure.

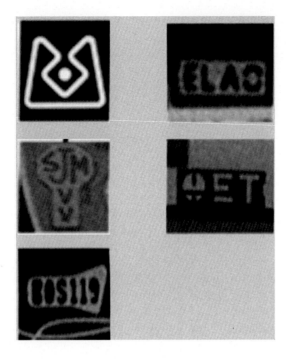

FIG. 2

Common manufacturer logos. Medtronic (*upper left*), Abbott (St. Jude Medical) (*middle left*), Boston Scientific (*lower left*), Sorin Ela (*upper right*), and Biotronic (*lower right*). These logos help to identify the pacemaker brand.

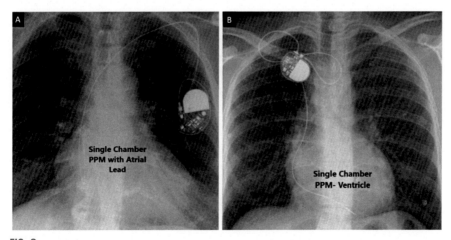

FIG. 3

Single-chamber pacemakers. Panel A: Single-chamber atrial pacemaker implanted via the left subclavian vein. Panel B: Single-chamber ventricular pacemaker in the right ventricle via the right subclavian vein.

Pacemaker lead types

Pacemaker generators transmit electrical activity to the heart via unipolar or bipolar leads (Fig. 4).

Leads reach the myocardium via endocardial (through venous system) or epicardial aspects (Fig. 5).

The type of fixation to the heart can be passive or active (Fig. 6). Pacemaker lead fixation in the heart is very important to avoid lead dislodgement and for better pacing and sensing thresholds.

Sometimes the atrial-sensing electrode is on the atrial aspect of the passive ventricular lead. In this model, lead configuration in the atrial level has the sensing with no pacing capability (Fig. 7).

In bipolar leads, there are two electrical strings, tip and ring electrodes and pacing or sensing modes could be bipolar or unipolar. In unipolar leads, the electrical circuit is between the tip of the lead and usually the generator body or other electronic structures (for example, unipolar pacing from tip of coronary sinus lead and an RV coil in defibrillator lead). In unipolar lead, if the operator accidently changes the unipolar pacing mode to a bipolar configuration, the pacing function will be lost. This issue in old unipolar implanted endocardial or epicardial leads is dangerous. This point is very important during pacemaker replacement. The electrical circuit is dependent on the contact between the generator and the pocket. We can see large pacing spikes in more ECG leads when the pacing mode is unipolar. In bipolar leads, the electrical circuit can be between two distinguished electrodes, tip and ring. We can change the pacing and sensing circuit from the bipolar mode to the unipolar mode (for example, between lead tip and generator). In well-known situations, such as cardiac defibrillators, only a bipolar-sensing pattern is acceptable and we cannot change it to a unipolar pattern to avoid electromagnetic interference.

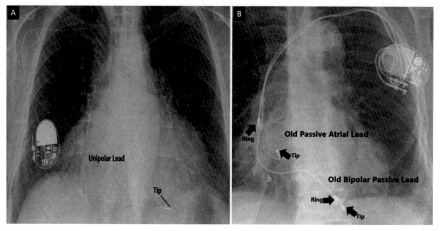

FIG. 4

Unipolar lead vs bipolar lead. Panel A: Unipolar ventricular lead. Note that there is no fixation screw. Passive fixation tines are not visible in chest radiograph (radiolucent). Panel B: Bipolar passive leads in the right atrial appendage and the right ventricular apex.

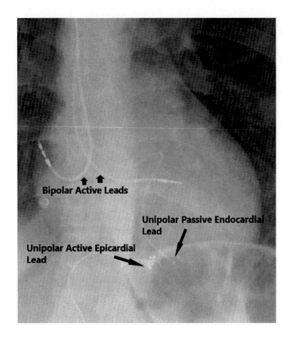

FIG. 5

Endocardial vs epicardial leads. Two active endocardial leads, one passive endocardial, and one active epicardial leads are shown. Lead diameters in endocardial vs epicardial leads can be compared.

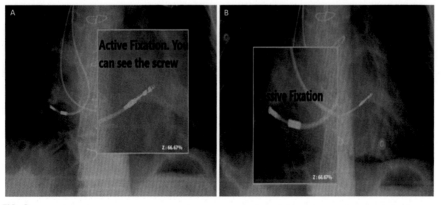

FIG. 6

Active fixation vs passive fixation leads. Panel A: Lead screwing in the myocardium for better adhesion. This form of fixation is called active fixation. Panel B: In passive fixation, a specific radiolucent structure in the lead helps for fixation into a trabeculated organ, such as an appendage in the right atrium or an apical portion of the right ventricle.

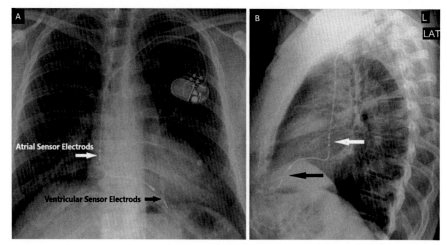

FIG. 7

Posteroanterior and lateral views of a single-lead dual-chamber pacemaker (so-called VDD pacemaker). The *white arrow* shows the atrial-sensing electrode, and the *black arrow* shows the ventricular-sensing and pacing electrode.

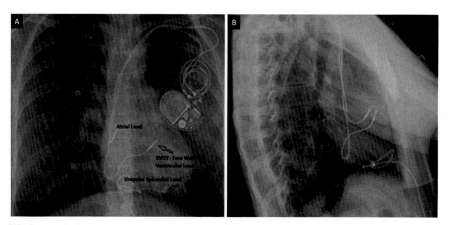

FIG. 8

Upgrading a single-chamber epicardial pacemaker to a dual-chamber endocardial pacemaker. The atrial lead is fixed in the right atrial appendage. It has a slight medial course on the posteroanterior view (Panel A), while on the lateral view, its location is anterior and forms a "J" loop (Panel B).

Pacing and sensing modalities are effective through the pacemaker lead tip and rarely, ring electrodes. These options are programmable through pacemaker analysis. The unipolar pacing circuit is larger than the bipolar pacing circuit; therefore, electromagnetic interference is more probable.

The atrial lead is usually fixed to the right atrium appendage or the interatrial septum (Fig. 8).

The usual location for RV lead fixation is at the RV apex or the septum (Fig. 9). RV septal pacing is noninferior to RV apical pacing for reverse left ventricular remodeling. A lateral view helps to differentiate the septal position from the anterior wall placement [4].

His bundle pacing is a new technology that helps to reduce the risk of pacing-induced cardiomyopathy (Fig. 10) [5]. This topic is covered in more detail in Chapter 6.

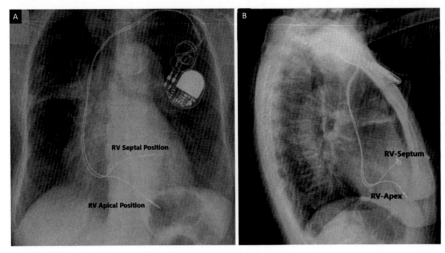

FIG. 9

Multifocal right ventricular (RV) pacing. Panel A: Two RV leads are implanted into the RV septum and the apex. Panel B: Both leads have an anterior course; however, the RV septal lead has upward orientation and the RV apical lead has downward orientation.

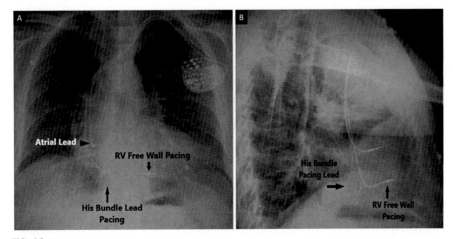

FIG. 10

A triple-chamber pacemaker with one atrial lead, one His pacing, and one right ventricular lead. Panel A: The His pacing lead is located near the tricuspid annulus and has a smaller diameter compared with the RV lead implanted in the anterior wall of right ventricle. The RV lead has more apical location compared with the His pacing lead. Panel B: These features are better illustrated in the lateral view.

Types of pacemaker lead connections to a generator

The ends of the pacemaker leads of today have an international standard shape (Fig. 11). Therefore, different traditional lead brands can connect to different generator brands. In very old lead types, the physician uses an adaptor to connect the lead to the new generator. The lead connection to the generator has been following international standards for years. If the lead is too old, an adapter is used to connect to the generator.

Endocardial pacemaker implantation in the prosthetic tricuspid valve

In patients with a metallic tricuspid valve, it is not possible to deploy a ventricular lead in the right ventricular chamber (Fig. 12).

Left ventricular stimulation via coronary sinus branches is a good option. Coronary sinus leads have different shapes. They can be unipolar or bipolar in structure. More details are provided in Chapter 4.

In patients with a prior transvenous pacemaker, cardiac surgeons can save RV transvenous leads during valve surgery (Fig. 13).

Pacemaker implantation in congenital heart disease

Vein access is usually from the left or right axillary veins or from the subclavian veins. These veins drain directly into the SVC and the right atrium (Fig. 14).

In a few patients, the left subclavian vein connects to the left SVC (Fig. 15).

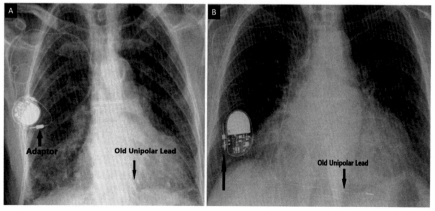

FIG. 11

Two currently available single-chamber pacemakers connected to two types of unipolar leads. Panel A: An old unipolar lead is connected to the pacemaker using an adapter (*thick black arrow*). Panel B: A newer unipolar lead is connected to the generator without an adaptor (*black long arrow*).

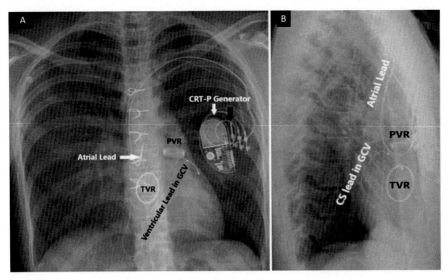

FIG. 12

Posteroanterior (A) and lateral (B) views of a triple-chamber pacemaker in a patient with prosthetic tricuspid (TVR) and pulmonic (PVR) valves. The atrial lead (*white arrow*) is implanted in the right atrial appendage, and the ventricular lead is placed via the great cardiac vein (GCV) in the anterior interventricular vein. A seal plug is inserted into the third empty connecting port of the generator (*black arrow*).

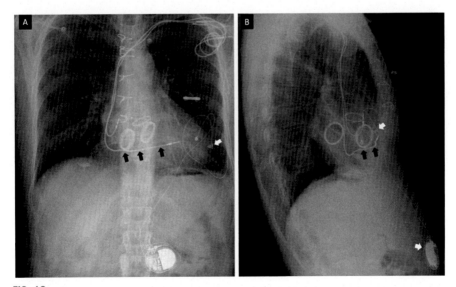

FIG. 13

Posteroanterior and lateral views of the retained right ventricular (RV) lead in a patient with a prosthetic tricuspid valve. Panel A: Retained RV lead (*black arrows*) outside the ring of the prosthetic tricuspid valve. RV lead course through the periphery of the prosthetic tricuspid valve is clearly shown in Panel B. The patient also has an epicardial lead connected to a single-chamber pacemaker implanted in the abdominal wall (*white arrows*).

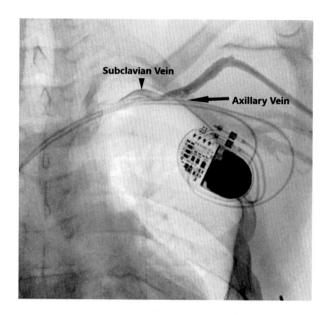

FIG. 14

Venogram showing dual-chamber pacemaker lead insertion via the left axillary and then the subclavian veins. These veins drain directly into the SVC and the right atrium.

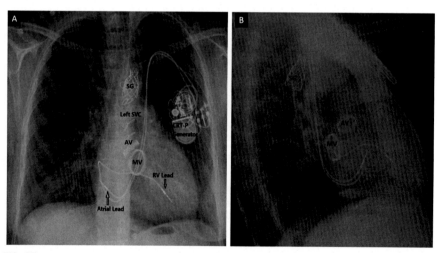

FIG. 15

Dual-chamber pacemaker implantation via a persistent left superior vena cava (SVC). Panel A: The right atrial and right ventricular (RV) leads are passed through the left side of the mediastinum via the left SVC rather than via the right SVC. Panel B: The right atrial and RV leads have a more posterior course compared with lead implantation via the right SVC. The patient also has a stent graft for aortic coarctation (SG) and prosthetic aortic (AV) and mitral valve (MV).

As endocardial leads function better than epicardial leads, there is a greater tendency to implant endocardial leads in patients. In congenital heart disease, great attention should be paid to the presence of intracardiac shunts and available venous pathways. The problem in the mentioned cases is an obstacle for implantation of pacemaker by endocardial method.

In patients with an intracardiac shunt, complex congenital heart disease, or obstructed vein access, the surgeon implants an epicardial lead. In many centers, surgeons implant epicardial leads for pacing in babies weighing less than 10 kg. The epicardial lead (Figs. 16 and 17) can be fixed on the heart via scrowing or suturing. The pacing threshold in suture-on leads is usually better than that in screw-in leads. Unipolar leads are more commonly used than bipolar epicardial leads (Fig. 17).

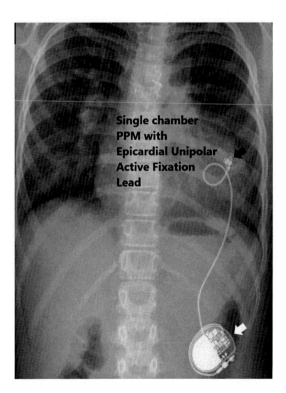

FIG. 16

Single-chamber pacemaker connected to an epicardial lead. The epicardial lead is unipolar and connected using a screw to the epicardial surface of the right ventricle (*black arrow*). The generator of the single-chamber pacemaker is placed within a pocket in the anterior abdominal wall (*white arrow*).

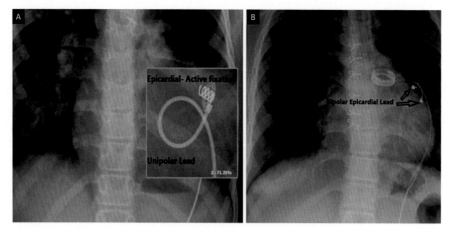

FIG. 17

Posteroanterior view of two single-chamber epicardial pacemakers. In Panel A, a unipolar epicardial lead is fixed via screwing. In Panel B, a bipolar epicardial lead is fixed via suturing.

References

[1] O. Aquilina, A brief history of cardiac pacing, Images Paediatr Cardiol 8 (2) (2006) 17–81.

[2] M.D. FranciscoLeyva, P.D. SeahNisam, M.D. Angelo Auricchio, PhD 20 years of cardiac resynchronization therapy, J Am Coll Cardiol 64 (10) (2014) 1047–1058.

[3] S. Jacob, M.A. Shahzad, R. Maheshwari, S.S. Panaich, R. Aravindhakshan, Cardiac rhythm device identification algorithm using X-rays: CaRDIA-X, Heart Rhythm 8 (2011) 915–922.

[4] C. Leclercq, N. Sadoul, L. Mont, P. Defaye, J. Osca, E. Mouton, R. Isnard, G. Habib, J. Zamorano, G. Derumeaux, I. Fernandez-Lozano, SEPTAL CRT Study Investigators, Comparison of right ventricular septal pacing and right ventricular apical pacing in patients receiving cardiac resynchronization therapy defibrillators: the SEPTAL CRT Study, Eur Heart J 37 (5) (2016) 473–483, https://doi.org/10.1093/eurheartj/ehv422.

[5] A.J.M. Lewis, P. Foley, Z. Whinnett, D. Keene, B. Chandrasekaran, His bundle pacing: a new strategy for physiological ventricular activation [published correction appears in J Am Heart Assoc. 2019 Jun 4;8(11):e002310], J Am Heart Assoc 8 (6) (2019), https://doi.org/10.1161/JAHA.118.010972, e010972.

Implantable cardioverter defibrillator devices

3

Farzad Kamali[a,b,*]

*aDepartment of Cardiac Electrophysiology, Rajaie Cardiovascular Medical and Research Center,
Iran University of Medical Sciences, Tehran, Iran*
*bCardiac Electrophysiology Research Center, Rajaie Cardiovascular Medical and Research
Center, Iran University of Medical Sciences, Tehran, Iran*
*Corresponding author: kamali.farzad@gmail.com

Key Points

- Every day, multiple implantable cardiac defibrillators (ICDs) are implanted for primary and secondary prevention of sudden cardiac death due to life-threatening arrhythmia. Chest radiography (CXR) is an important diagnostic in the identification of these devices.
- The main components of the ICD system include a pulse generator, defibrillation coils, and pace-sense electrodes. All these components are detectable by CXR.
- In ICD leads, the shock coils are radiopaque and easily distinguishable from pacemaker leads.

Introduction

One of the most effective treatments for life-threatening cardiac arrhythmia is implantable cardioverter defibrillators (ICD), which have been developed over the last few decades. Chest radiography (CXR) plays an important role in assessing the position and complications of cardiac implantable devices after initial implantation and during follow-up [1]. In this chapter, our goal in is to familiarize cardiovascular residents with both normal and abnormal radiographic appearances of ICDs.

Indications for ICD

The main indications for ICD implantation include secondary prevention and primary prevention.

Secondary prevention

An ICD is the first-line treatment option for secondary prevention of SCD due to VF or sustained hemodynamically unstable VT in patients with structural heart disease and in those with idiopathic VT/VF and congenital channelopathies. Sustained hemodynamically stable VT in patients with structural heart disease is also an indication for secondary ICD implantation.

Primary prevention

For patients with ischemic and nonischemic cardiomyopathy, LVEF$\leq$35%, and NYHA functional class II or III, ICD implantation for primary prevention of SCD is recommended.

ICDs for primary prevention are also recommended for patients with ischemic cardiomyopathy (at least 40 days after myocardial infarction and more than 3 months following revascularization), LVEF$\leq$30%, and NYHA functional class I.

Contraindications for ICD

In the following conditions, ICD implantation is not recommended:

- For primary prevention of SCD within 40 days after MI.
- For patients with NYHA functional class IV heart failure that is refractory to medical treatment and for candidates not suitable for transplantation or CRT (cardiac resynchronization therapy).
- For patients with life expectancy of not more than 1 year with an acceptable functional status.
- For patients with incessant VT/VF, ICD implantation is not recommended without arrhythmia control.

ICD components

The main components of an ICD system include (1) a pulse generator, (2) defibrillation coils, and (3) pacing/sensing electrodes (Figs. 1 and 2).

A pulse generator contains electronic circuitry, high-voltage capacitors, and a battery. Generators are usually implanted subcutaneously in the infraclavicular region of the anterior chest wall. For implantation of a generator, the left pectoral is preferable to the right pectoral because the defibrillation vector between the distal coil and the generator can cover more of the left ventricle.

ICD leads have both sensing/pacing and defibrillation functions simultaneously.

The sensing/pacing function is possible with the distal electrode at the tip of the ICD lead and with a second ring electrode several milliliters back from the tip (true bipolar ICD lead). True bipolar ICD leads are dedicated to bipolar sensing and pacing between the tip and ring electrodes. Integrated ICD leads have only a tip electrode, so sensing and pacing occurs between the tip and the distal defibrillation electrode (Fig. 3).

Defibrillation electrodes or shock coils are graphically opaque and thick and are easily distinguishable from pacemaker leads. The RV lead in ICDs has one or two defibrillation electrodes or coils. In single-coil ICD leads, the defibrillation electrode is located in the right ventricle (RV), while dual-coil ICD leads have a second proximal defibrillation electrode at the brachiocephalic vein–superior vena cava junction.

In the past, the epicardial ICD system and epicardial patches were used for defibrillation (Fig. 4). Implantation of epicardial defibrillation patches required a left thoracotomy or a midline sternotomy.

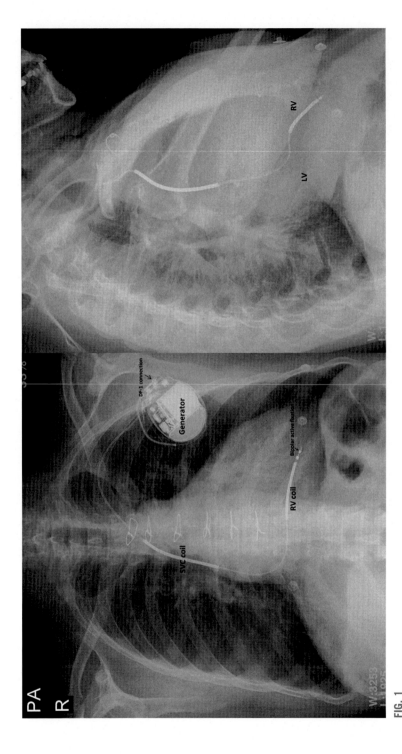

FIG. 1

CXR in the posteroanterior (*left image*) and lateral (*right image*) views shows a single-chamber ICD (ICD-VR). The pulse generator is positioned subcutaneously in the left pectoral region. The extensions of the connector pins beyond the set screw are normal, radiographically. The dual-coil ICD lead (DF-1 type) with active fixation is placed at the RV apex. The proximal shock coil is located at the left brachiocephalic–superior vena cava junction, while the distal shock coil is in the right ventricle (RV). The type of ICD lead connection to the generator is IS-1/DF-1. Poststernotomy suture is observed on the X-ray. Lead integrity is normal. Gross complications are not visible.

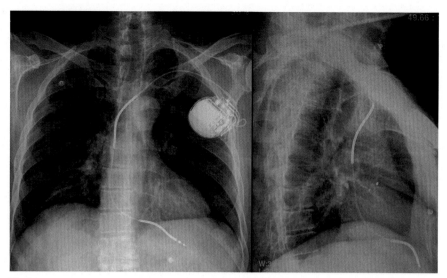

FIG. 2

CXR in the posteroanterior and lateral views shows a single-chamber ICD (ICD-VR). The pulse generator is positioned subcutaneously in the left pectoral region. The extensions of the connector pins beyond the set screw are normal, radiographically. The dual-coil ICD lead (DF-1 type) with active fixation is placed at the RV apex. The proximal shock coil is located at the left brachiocephalic–superior vena cava junction, while the distal shock coil is in the RV. Lead integrity is normal. Gross complications are not visible.

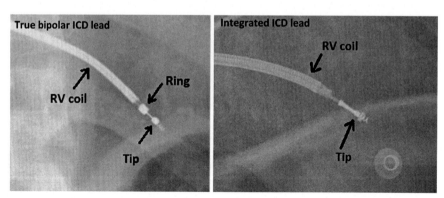

FIG. 3

Left image shows a true bipolar ICD lead (dedicated lead). In a true bipolar lead, the sensing/pacing function is possible between the tip and ring electrodes, while in an integrated ICD lead (*right image*), sensing/pacing occurs between the lead tip and RV defibrillation coil.

Types of ICDs

Just like pacemakers, ICDs have three types based on the number of cardiac chambers where the leads are implanted. Single-chamber ICDs have only an RV shock lead. Dual-chamber ICDs have right atrial (RA) and RV shock leads (Figs. 5 and 6).

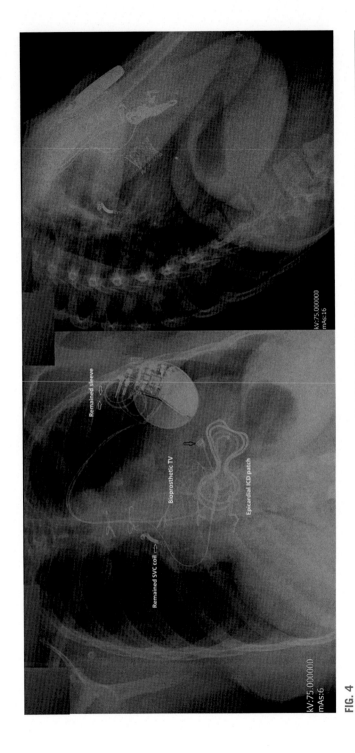

FIG. 4

CXR in the posteroanterior and lateral views shows an ICD with epicardial patch system. A unipolar screw-in RV lead (*black arrow*) is also implanted epicardially and connected to the ICD generator in the left pectoral region. Remains of the previous endocardial ICD lead, which was extracted surgically, are shown in white arrows on the CXR. A bioprosthetic heart valve in the tricuspid position and poststernotomy suture are visible.

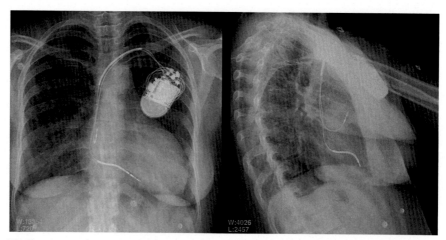

FIG. 5

CXR in the posteroanterior and lateral views shows a dual-chamber ICD (ICD-DR). The pulse generator is positioned subcutaneously in the left pectoral region. The extensions of the connector pins beyond the set screw are normal. The dual-coil ICD lead (DF-1 type) with active fixation is placed in the RV interventricular septum. The proximal shock coil is located at the left subclavian–brachiocephalic junction, while the distal shock coil is in the RV. An endocardial bipolar atrial lead with an active fixation correctly placed is at the right atrial appendage with a "J-loop" appearance. The integrity of leads is normal.

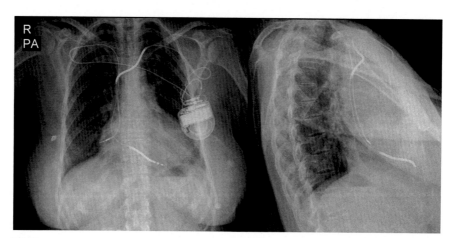

FIG. 6

CXR in the posteroanterior and lateral views shows a dual-chamber ICD (ICD-DR). The ICD generator is positioned in the left pectoral region. An endocardial dual-coil ICD lead (DF-1 type) with active fixation is placed near the RV apex through the left subclavian vein. The proximal shock coil is located at the subclavian–brachiocephalic junction, while the distal shock coil is in the RV. An endocardial bipolar atrial lead with active fixation is placed at the RA free wall through the right subclavian vein and is then tunneled subcutaneously across the midline to the generator in the left pectoral region.

Cardiac resynchronization therapy defibrillator (CTR−D) devices have RA, RV, (shock lead), and left ventricular (LV) leads. LV leads are positioned into the free-wall cardiac veins through the coronary sinus (see the chapter "Cardiac resynchronization Therapy").

Types of ICD lead connections to a generator

There are two types of ICD lead connections to a generator, namely, DF-1 and DF-4 (Figs. 1, 7, and 8).

The IS-1/DF-1 ICD lead has bifurcated (in single coil) or a trifurcated (in dual coil) header connector pins. The sense/pace portion of the lead is terminated with an IS-1 pin, and the high-voltage coils are terminated with pins of their respective defibrillators. The DF-4 leads have only one plug providing four poles (two distal poles for sense/pace and two proximal poles for defibrillator coils).

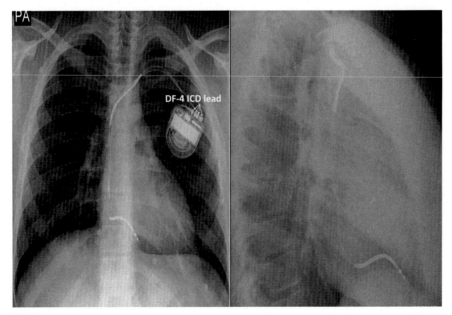

FIG. 7

CXR in the posteroanterior and lateral views shows a dual-chamber ICD (ICD-DR). The pulse generator is positioned subcutaneously in the left pectoral region. The extensions of the connector pins beyond the set screw are normal. The dual-coil ICD lead (DF-4) with active fixation is placed in the right interventricular septum. An endocardial bipolar atrial lead with an active fixation correctly placed is at the right atrial appendage with a "J-loop" appearance. As shown on the CXR (white arrows), the DF-4 leads have only one plug providing four poles (two distal poles for sense/pace and two proximal poles for defibrillation coils).

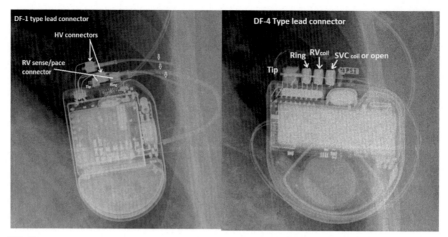

FIG. 8

Magnified images of the two types of ICD lead connectors. The *left image* shows a DF-1 type ICD lead with a trifurcated header connector pin. DF-4 type ICD leads (*right image*) have only one plug providing four poles (two distal poles for sense/pace and two proximal poles for defibrillator coils).

ICD in patients with a left ventricular assist device

A left ventricular assist device (LVAD) is an electromechanical pump that is used in patients with end-stage heart failure for assisting cardiac circulation. The presence of ICDs is common among patients referred for LVAD therapy (Fig. 9). ICDs can be implanted before or after LVAD.

Inadvertent ICD lead placement

The ideal position of an ICD lead is at the RV apex, but in certain circumstances (such as a low sensing threshold at the RV apex), the ICD lead may be placed in other sites such as the RV upper septum (Fig. 10) or the right ventricular outflow tract. On a frontal radiograph, the tip of the RV lead should be located to the left of the spine, while on the lateral view, it should be located anteriorly.

Inadvertent ICD lead placement into other cardiac chambers, such as LV and great cardiac vein, is rare (Fig. 11), but may occur if the operator is inattentive during the procedure. Careful fluoroscopy of the leads in multiple views prevents this complication.

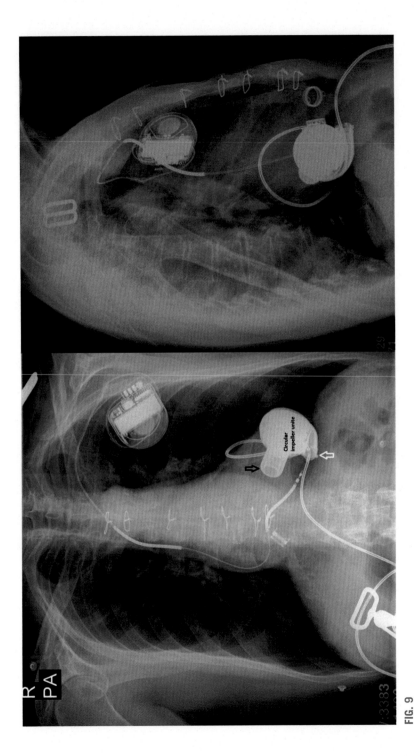

FIG. 9

CXR in the posteroanterior and lateral views shows a single-chamber ICD (ICD-VR). The pulse generator is positioned subcutaneously in the left pectoral region. The extension of the connector pin beyond the set screw is normal, radiographically. The dual-coil ICD lead (DF-4) with active fixation is placed at the RV apex. The proximal shock coil is located at the left brachiocephalic–superior vena cava junction, while the distal shock coil is in the right ventricular. Lead integrity is normal. A HeartWare left ventricular assist device (LVAD) is situated in a normal position. Note that the HeartWare LVAD has a round-shaped impeller unit and an inflow cannula (*black arrow*) and an outflow cannula (*white arrow*).

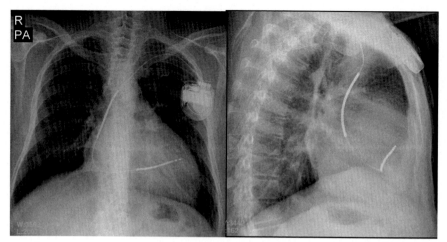

FIG. 10

CXR in the posteroanterior and lateral views shows a single-chamber ICD (ICD-VR). The pulse generator is positioned subcutaneously in the left pectoral region. The extension of the connector pin beyond the set screw is normal. The dual-coil ICD lead (DF-4) with active fixation is placed in the RV upper septum. The proximal shock coil is located at the left brachiocephalic–superior vena cava junction, while the distal shock coil is in the RV. Severe cardiomegaly and biventricular enlargement are noted.

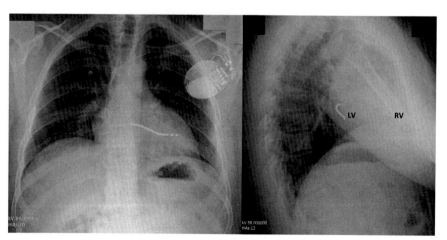

FIG. 11

CXR in the posteroanterior and lateral views shows a single-chamber ICD (ICD-VR). The pulse generator is positioned subcutaneously in the left pectoral region. The extensions of the connector pins beyond the set screw are normal, radiographically. On posteroanterior chest radiograph, the ICD lead (single-coil DF-4 type) appeared to be positioned in the proper site in the RV mid-septum. The lateral view shows a posterior diversion of the ICD lead. Inadvertent left-sided ventricular lead placement through a patent foramen ovale was confirmed by transesophageal echocardiography.

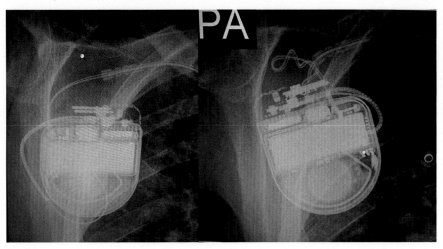

FIG. 12

A magnified X-ray of an ICD generator is shown at the time of implantation (left radiograph) and 3 months after implantation (right radiograph) in an elderly man, who had presented with an ICD lead dislodgement. The ICD lead tangling and rotation of the generator are seen on the right-side radiograph. These radiographic findings suggest Twiddler's syndrome and rotation and manipulation of the generator along its longitudinal axis.

Twiddler's syndrome and reel syndrome

Twiddler's syndrome is an uncommon condition that occurs when a patient manipulates and rotates a device generator. Continued rotation of a generator can cause lead dislodgment and coiling of leads around the generator. Rotation of the generator may occur either along its longitudinal (Fig. 12) or transverse axis. Reel syndrome is a variant of Twiddler's syndrome in which the leads are wrapped around the generator along its transverse or horizontal axis [2].

References

[1] A.L. Aguilera, Y.V. Volokhina, K.L. Fisher, Radilogy of cardiac conduction devices: a comprehensive review, Radiographics 31 (6) (2011) 1669–1682, https://doi.org/10.1148/rg.
[2] A. Carnero-Varo, M. Pérez-Paredes, J.A. Ruiz-Ros, D. Giménez-Cervantes, F.R. Martínez-Corbalán, T. Cubero-López, P. Jara-Pérez, Reel syndrome, Circulation 100 (1999) e45–e46, https://doi.org/10.1161/01.CIR.100.8.e45.

Cardiac resynchronization therapy devices

4

Majid Haghjoo[a,b,*]

[a]*Department of Cardiac Electrophysiology, Rajaie Cardiovascular Medical and Research Center,*
Iran University of Medical Sciences, Tehran, Iran
[b]*Cardiac Electrophysiology Research Center, Rajaie Cardiovascular Medical and Research*
Center, Iran University of Medical Sciences, Tehran, Iran
*Corresponding author: majid.haghjoo@gmail.com

Key Points

- The assessment of a cardiac resynchronization therapy (CRT) device on a chest radiograph is not different from other cardiac implantable electronic devices.
- As the shock coils are radiopaque, they can be readily identified on a chest radiograph, enabling a CRT defibrillator to be differentiated from a CRT pacemaker.
- Lateral views allow a distinction to be made between an anteriorly placed right ventricle lead and a posteriorly coursed left ventricle lead.

Introduction

Cardiac resynchronization therapy (CRT) devices are used for treating patients with drug-refractory symptomatic heart failure [1]. A cardiac resynchronization device can be a defibrillator (CRT−D) or a pacemaker (CRT−P). Defibrillator form of the CRT has the capability to deliver synchronized or unsynchronized shocks to terminate life-threatening ventricular arrhythmias; therefore, it needs a triple-chamber defibrillator generator and an RV lead with shock coils. However, a CRT-P device uses a triple-chamber pacemaker generator and a sense/pace RV lead without shock coils.

CRT components

All CRT devices consist of a generator (defibrillator or pacemaker) and three leads: a right atrium (RA) lead, a right ventricle (RV) lead, and a left ventricular (LV) lead. CRT devices have the same types of RA and LV leads, but they use different types of generators and RV leads (Fig. 1).

Radiographic Atlas of Cardiac Implantable Electronic Devices. https://doi.org/10.1016/B978-0-323-84753-7.00004-2

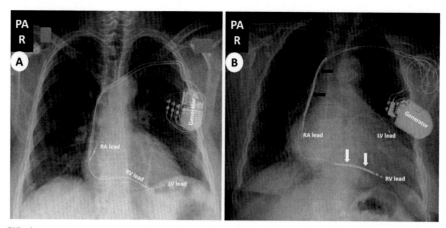

FIG. 1

Posteroanterior (PA) chest radiographs showing two kinds of cardiac resynchronization therapy (CRT) devices. Panel A shows a pacemaker-only CRT device (CRT–P). There are three leads, including a right atrial (RA) lead in the right atrial appendage (RAA), a right ventricular (RV) pacemaker lead at the RV apex, and a bipolar left ventricular (LV) lead in the posterolateral cardiac vein. Panel B shows a CRT device with defibrillation capability (CRT–D) with an RA lead in the RAA, an RV defibrillator lead in the low septum, and an LV lead in the anterolateral cardiac vein. Note that RA and LV leads are similar in both devices; however, the RV lead in CRT-D has shock coils in the superior vena cava (*black arrow*) and the RV portion of the lead (*white arrow*) and its generator is larger mainly due to the presence of the capacitor.

1. *RA lead*: The RA sense/pace lead is located in the atrial appendage. This lead first travels inferiorly into the right atrium and then turns upward and anteriorly where it is anchored within the trabeculae of the atrial appendage. The same types of sense/pace RA leads are used in CRT-P and CRT-D devices (Fig. 1).
2. *RV lead*: The tip of the RV lead is positioned at the apex of the right ventricle, which is located to the left of the spine on a posteroanterior view of the chest radiograph (CXR) and anteriorly on a lateral view (Fig. 1). However, an RV lead can be implanted in a different part of the septum from low to high septum (Figs. 2–4). The RV lead in CRT-D has one or two coils (Fig. 5). As these shock coils are radiopaque, they can be readily identified on a chest X-ray, enabling a CRT-D to be differentiated from a CRT-P (Fig. 1).
3. *LV lead*: The LV lead travels through the RA and the coronary sinus (CS) and is finally positioned into free-wall cardiac veins (Figs. 6–8). Lateral views allow a distinction to be made between an anteriorly placed RV lead and a posteriorly coursed LV lead [2]. The same types of sense/pace LV leads are used in CRT-P and CRT-D devices. Different types of LV leads are available for implantation, including unipolar, bipolar, or quadripolar leads (Figs. 9–11).

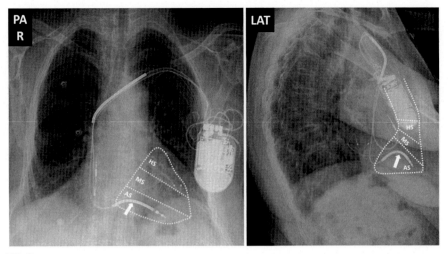

FIG. 2

Posteroanterior (PA) and lateral (LAT) chest radiographs showing a cardiac resynchronization therapy device with a right atrial lead in the right atrial appendage and a left ventricular lead in the lateral cardiac vein. Note that the right ventricular shock lead (*white arrow*) is implanted in the apical part of the interventricular septum (apicoseptum, AS).

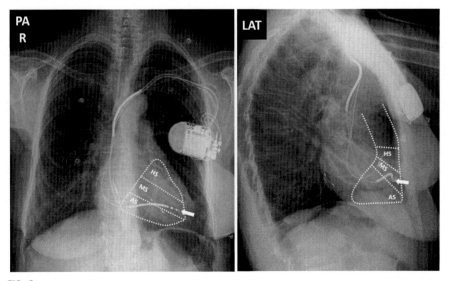

FIG. 3

Posteroanterior (PA) and lateral (LAT) chest radiographs showing a cardiac resynchronization therapy device with a right atrial lead in the right atrial appendage and a left ventricular lead in the lateral cardiac vein. Note that the right ventricular shock lead (*white arrow*) is implanted in the middle part of the interventricular septum (mid-septum, MS).

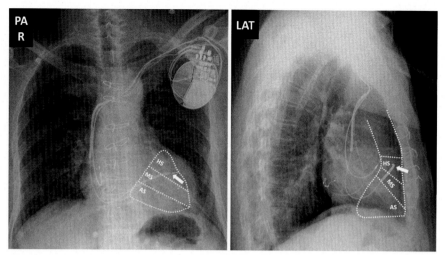

FIG. 4

Posteroanterior (PA) and lateral (LAT) chest radiographs showing a cardiac resynchronization therapy device with a right atrial lead in the right atrial appendage and a left ventricular lead in the lateral coronary vein. Note that the right ventricular shock lead (*white arrow*) is implanted in the high septum (HS).

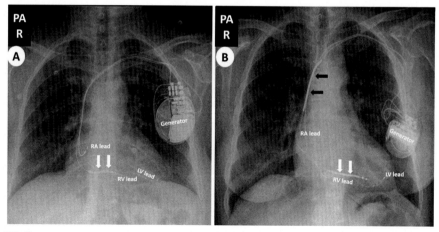

FIG. 5

Posteroanterior (PA) chest radiographs of two cardiac resynchronization therapy systems with defibrillation capability (CRT–D). In Panel A, the right ventricular (RV) lead has only one shock coil in the RV part of the lead (*white arrow*). In Panel B, the RV lead has two coils, one in the superior vena cava (*black arrow*) part of the lead (SVC coil) and the other coil in the RV part of the lead (*white arrow*).

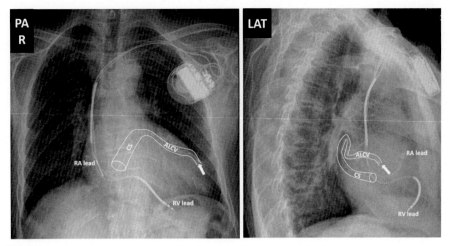

FIG. 6

Posteroanterior (PA) and lateral (LAT) chest radiographs showing a cardiac resynchronization therapy device with a right atrial (RA) lead in the right atrial appendage and a right ventricular (RV) lead at the right ventricular apex. In this case, the left ventricular lead (*white arrow*) is implanted via the coronary sinus (CS) in the anterolateral cardiac vein (ALCV).

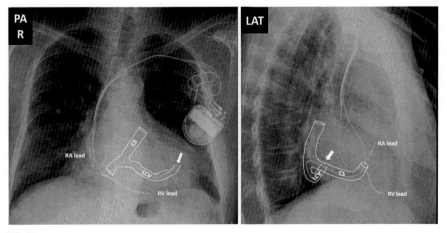

FIG. 7

Posteroanterior (PA) and lateral (LAT) chest radiographs showing a cardiac resynchronization therapy device with a right atrial (RA) lead in the right atrial free wall and a right ventricular (RV) lead at the right ventricular apex. In this case, the left ventricular lead (white arrow) is implanted via the coronary sinus (CS) in the lateral cardiac vein (LCV).

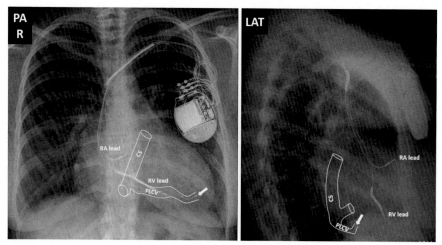

FIG. 8

Posteroanterior (PA) and lateral (LAT) chest radiographs showing a cardiac resynchronization therapy device with a right atrial (RA) lead in the right atrial appendage and a right ventricular (RV) lead in the low septum. In this case, the left ventricular lead (white arrow) is implanted via the coronary sinus (CS) in the posterolateral cardiac vein (PLCV).

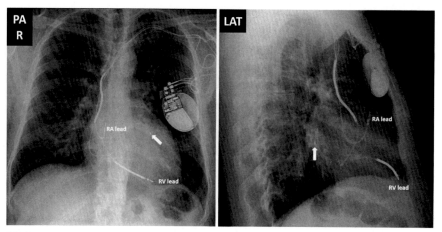

FIG. 9

Posteroanterior (PA) and lateral (LAT) chest radiographs showing a cardiac resynchronization therapy device with a right atrial (RA) lead in the right atrial appendage and a right ventricular (RV) lead at the right ventricular apex. In this case, a unipolar left ventricular lead (white arrow) is implanted in the anterolateral cardiac vein.

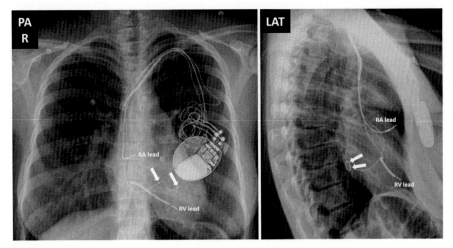

FIG. 10

Posteroanterior (PA) and lateral (LAT) chest radiographs showing a cardiac resynchronization therapy device with a right atrial (RA) lead in the right atrial appendage and a right ventricular (RV) lead at the right ventricular apex. In this case, a bipolar left ventricular lead (white arrow) is implanted in the lateral cardiac vein.

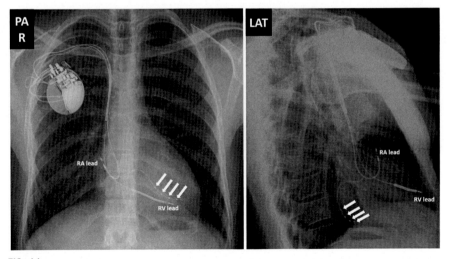

FIG. 11

Posteroanterior (PA) and lateral (LAT) chest radiographs showing a cardiac resynchronization therapy device with a right atrial (RA) lead in the right atrial free wall and a right ventricular (RV) lead at the right ventricular apex. In this case, a quadripolar left ventricular lead is implanted in the lateral cardiac vein.

Coronary sinus venography

CRT implants can be complex and more time-consuming than dual-chamber devices mainly because of an LV lead implant. Before an LV lead implant, it is necessary to cannulate the CS. The CS is located at the base of the right atrium above the tricuspid annulus. Next, it is necessary to perform an occlusive CS venogram in the antero-posterior (AP) and left anterior oblique (LAO) views to visualize the available veins branching off of the CS (Fig. 12–15). These venograms are performed to better understand whether the veins are located in the lateral or anterior sections of the heart.

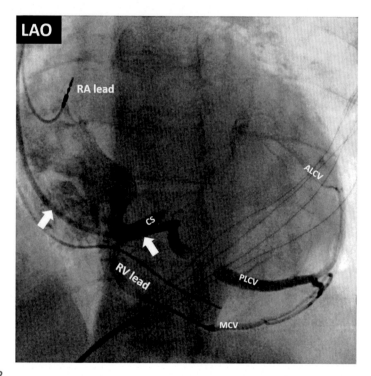

FIG. 12

An occlusive coronary sinus (CS) venogram in the left anterior oblique (LAO) view, showing the available veins branching off of the CS. Right atrial (RA) and right ventricular (RV) defibrillator leads are already implanted. A long sheath for venography and left ventricular lead delivery is placed within the CS (white arrow). Venogram shows one small anterolateral cardiac vein (ALCV) on top of the heart silhouette, then a sizable posterolateral cardiac vein (PLCV), and finally a middle cardiac vein (MCV) at the bottom.

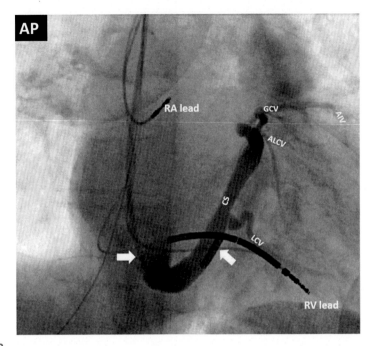

FIG. 13

An occlusive coronary sinus (CS) venogram in the anteroposterior (AP) view, showing the available veins branching off of the CS. Right atrial (RA) and right ventricular (RV) defibrillator leads are already implanted. A long sheath for venography and left ventricular lead delivery is placed within the CS (*white arrow*). Venogram shows CS continuation known as the great cardiac vein (GCV), the small anterior interventricular vein (AIV), and the small branching anterolateral cardiac vein (ALCV) on top of the heart silhouette, and then a sizable and tortuous lateral cardiac vein (LCV).

LV lead locations

LV leads are implanted in one of the free-wall draining coronary veins, including the posterolateral cardiac vein, the lateral cardiac vein, or the anterolateral cardiac vein. The middle cardiac vein and the anterior interventricular vein are not recommended for LV lead implantation because of septal stimulation (Figs. 16 and 17).

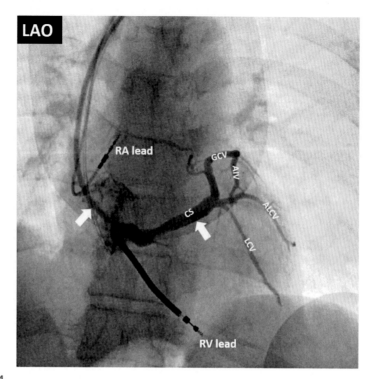

FIG. 14

An occlusive coronary sinus (CS) venogram in the left anterior oblique (LAO) view showing the available veins branching off of the CS. Right atrial (RA) and right ventricular (RV) defibrillator leads are already implanted. A long sheath for venography and left ventricular lead delivery is placed within the CS (*white arrow*). Venogram shows the CS, the great cardiac vein (GCV), and its continuation known as the anterior interventricular vein (AIV). The anterolateral cardiac vein (ALCV) and the lateral cardiac vein (LCV) stem from a common origin.

CRT in patients with congenital heart disease

The congenital heart disease (CHD) population has a high prevalence of heart failure during late follow-up, and this is a major cause of mortality. CRT may help to improve the clinical outcome of CHD patients with refractory HF. LV lead implantation would be very challenging in patients with congenitally corrected transposition of the great arteries (Fig. 18).

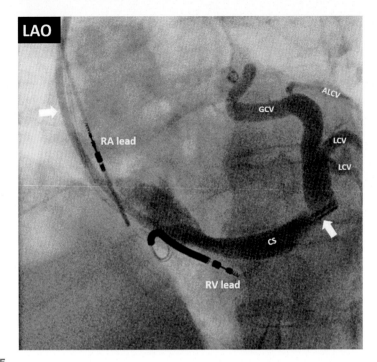

FIG. 15

An occlusive coronary sinus (CS) venogram in the left anterior oblique (LAO) view showing the available veins branching off of the CS. Right atrial (RA) and right ventricular (RV) defibrillator leads are already implanted. A long sheath for venography and left ventricular lead delivery is placed within the CS (white arrow). Venogram shows the CS, the great cardiac vein (GCV), the small anterolateral cardiac vein (ALCV), and branching sizable lateral cardiac vein (LCV).

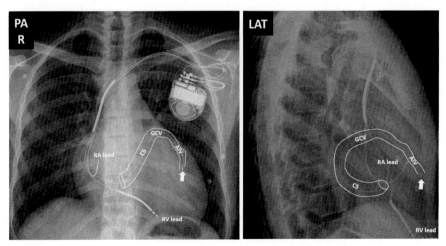

FIG. 16

Posteroanterior (PA) and lateral (LAT) chest radiographs showing a cardiac resynchronization therapy device with a right atrial (RA) lead in the right atrial appendage and a right ventricular (RV) lead at the right ventricular apex. In this case, the left ventricular lead (white arrow) is implanted in the anterior interventricular vein (AIV).

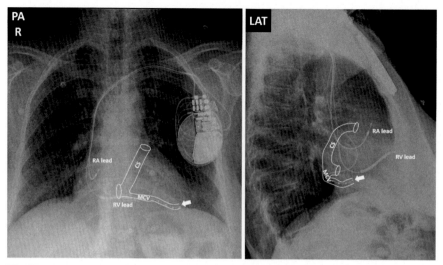

FIG. 17

Posteroanterior (PA) and lateral (LAT) chest radiographs showing a cardiac resynchronization therapy device with a right atrial (RA) lead in the right atrial appendage and a right ventricular (RV) lead in the mid-septal area. In this case, the left ventricular lead (*white arrow*) is implanted in the middle cardiac vein (MCV).

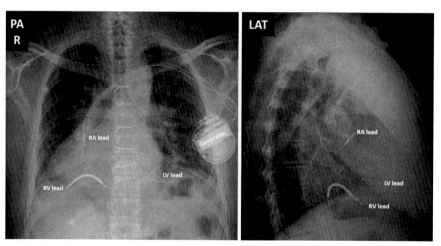

FIG. 18

Posteroanterior (PA) and lateral (LAT) chest radiographs showing a cardiac resynchronization therapy device in a patient with congenitally corrected transposition of great arteries (CCTGA). Note that right atrial (RA) and right ventricular (RV) leads are located in the right side of the thoracic vertebrae and the left ventricular (LV) lead on the left side. In the CCTGA setting, the PA view shows a better separation of the RV and LV leads compared with the LAT view (reverse that in a normal heart anatomy).

CRT in patients with a left ventricular assist device

Up to 30% of patients with HF failed to benefit from CRT. A left ventricular assist device (LVAD) supports ventricular pumping via mechanical unloading for a weakened heart. Therefore, it is not unusual to see HF patients having both CRT and LVAD (Fig. 19).

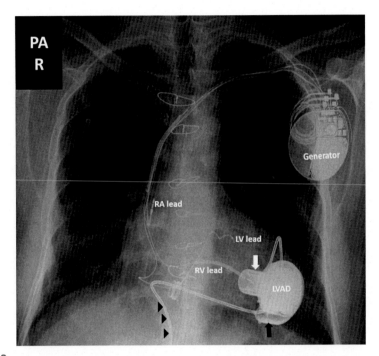

FIG. 19

Posteroanterior (PA) chest radiographs showing a cardiac resynchronization therapy device in a patient with a left ventricular assist device (LVAD). Note that the LVAD has an inflow (*white arrow*), an outflow (*black arrow*), and drive line (*black arrowheads*).

Combined endocardial–epicardial CRT

The coronary sinus can be difficult to cannulate in the case of an atretic vein or, more commonly, valves located over the ostium. Epicardial leads can be placed with a limited thoracotomy approach when the operator is unable to access the coronary sinus or find a suitable branch (Figs. 20 and 21).

CRT in patients with a prosthetic heart valve

Valvular heart disease may result in left ventricular dysfunction. Therefore, it is not unusual to see CXRs with CRT devices and prosthetic heart valves (Fig. 22).

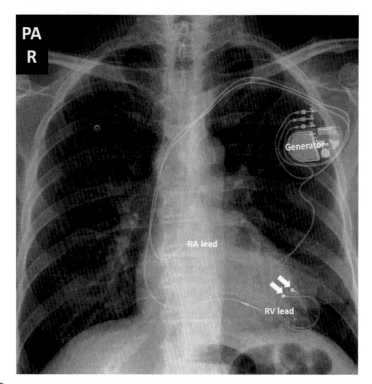

FIG. 20

Posteroanterior (PA) chest radiographs showing a cardiac resynchronization therapy pacemaker (CRT–P) device with right atrial (RA) and right ventricular (RV) leads implanted transvenously. Note that a bipolar suture-on left ventricular (LV) lead (*white arrows*) is implanted epicardially due to the absence of a proper vein and is tunneled subcutaneously and attached to a CRT-P generator.

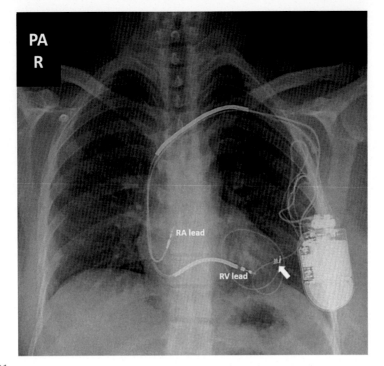

FIG. 21

Posteroanterior (PA) chest radiographs showing a cardiac resynchronization therapy defibrillator (CRT–D) device with right atrial (RA) and right ventricular (RV) leads implanted transvenously. Note that a screw-in left ventricular (LV) lead (*white arrow*) is implanted epicardially due to the absence of a proper vein and is tunneled subcutaneously and attached to a CRT-D generator.

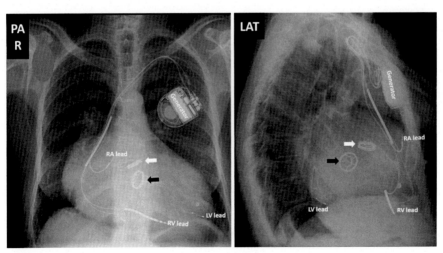

FIG. 22

Posteroanterior (PA) and lateral (LAT) chest radiographs showing a cardiac resynchronization therapy device in a patient with aortic and mitral prostheses. Note that the mitral prosthesis (*black arrow*) is directed toward the cardiac apex, and the aortic prosthesis (*white arrow*) is directed toward the aortic root.

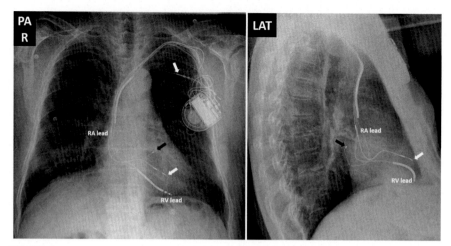

FIG. 23

Posteroanterior (PA) and lateral (LAT) chest radiographs showing a cardiac resynchronization therapy device with dislodged right atrial (RA) and left ventricular (LV) leads. Note that the right ventricular (RV) defibrillator lead is in the correct position within the RV. The LV lead (*black arrow*) is dislocated into the coronary sinus, and the active fixation RA lead is detached from the right atrial appendage and has lost its "J–curve." The terminal pin and distal electrode of the abandoned RV lead is shown by a *white arrow*.

LV lead dislodgement

Left ventricular lead dislodgement is underreported in the literature, being at least 10% at 1-year follow-ups. It occurs more frequently in the coronary veins close to the CS ostium and an upward course and in veins with a flat take-off at a > 80 degree angle from the CS (Fig. 23).

References

[1] W.T. Abraham, W.G. Fisher, A.L. Smith, D.B. Delurgio, A.R. Leon, E. Loh, D.Z. Kocovic, M. Packer, A.L. Clavell, D.L. Hayes, M. Ellestad, R.J. Trupp, J. Underwood, F. Pickering, C. Truex, P. McAtee, J. Messenger, MIRACLE Study Group, Multicenter InSync randomized clinical evaluation. Cardiac resynchronization in chronic heart failure, N Engl J Med 346 (24) (2002) 1845.
[2] A.L. Aguilera, Y.V. Volokhina, K.L. Fisher, Radiography of cardiac conduction devices: a comprehensive review, Radiographics 31 (2011) 1669–1682.

CIED complications

Amir Farjam Fazelifar[a,b,*]

[a]*Department of Cardiac Electrophysiology, Rajaie Cardiovascular Medical and Research Center,*
Iran University of Medical Sciences, Tehran, Iran
[b]*Cardiac Electrophysiology Research Center, Rajaie Cardiovascular Medical and Research*
Center, Iran University of Medical Sciences, Tehran, Iran
Corresponding author: fazelifar.academic@gmail.com

Key Points

- Chest radiography (CXR) is an important tool to detect early and late complications of cardiac implantable electronic device (CIED) implantations.
- Early and late CIED complications that are detectable with routine CXR include pneumothorax, hemothorax, lead perforation, lead dislodgment, lead fracture, and loose connection.
- Chest radiography also plays an important role in assessment of therapeutic interventions, such as chest tube insertion, lead revision, or lead reconnection.

Introduction

Cardiac implantable electronic device (CIED) implantation is an invasive procedure. Vein puncture for lead implantation may injure the lung or the vessels. Although many pacemaker malfunctions are detectable by device programming, chest radiography (CXR) is an important tool for differentiating between CIED complications.

It has been a standard practice to assess the lead position in CXR images taken 1 day after the procedure. The purpose of postprocedure CXR is to first rule out early complications, including pneumothorax and hemothorax, and then to evaluate the adequacy of the lead position and provide a reference for future comparisons. Chest radiography images can also help to detect late complications, such as lead fracture, perforation, and dislodgement.

In this chapter, we present clear images of the early and late complications of CIED implantations, which are detectable by posteroanterior (PA) and lateral views of routine CXRs.

Radiographic Atlas of Cardiac Implantable Electronic Devices. https://doi.org/10.1016/B978-0-323-84753-7.00005-4

Pneumothorax and hemothorax

Pneumothorax and hemothorax are early complications occurring after device implantation. Pneumothorax may complicate implantation of any kind of CIEDs, including pacemakers, defibrillators, or biventricular devices (Figs. 1–3).

Sometimes patients are totally asymptomatic, and complications can only be observed during a routine posteroanterior (PA) view (Fig. 4). In these cases, we occasionally need to take magnified images from the lung apex to reveal the pneumothorax line. In asymptomatic patients (the interpleural distance at the level of the hilum is less than 2cm), we can manage pneumothorax without inserting a chest tube. In these patients, serial CXRs help to follow the pneumothorax resolution or detect the progressive increase in the amount of air accumulation.

In case of chest tube insertion, CXRs are the diagnostic images of choice to evaluate the adequacy of air and fluid drainage (Fig. 5).

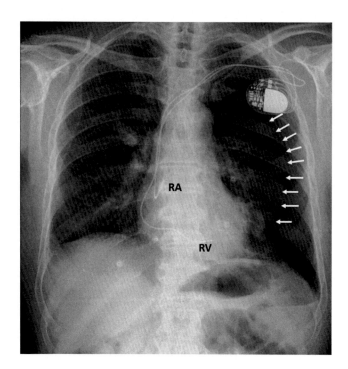

FIG. 1

Severe pneumothorax in a patient with a dual-chamber pacemaker. The right atrial (RA) lead was implanted in the right atrial appendage and the right ventricular (RV) lead in the low interventricular septum. *White arrows* show the line between the collapsed left lung and the ribcage in a posteroanterior view. Note that there is no lung vasculature between this line and the ribcage.

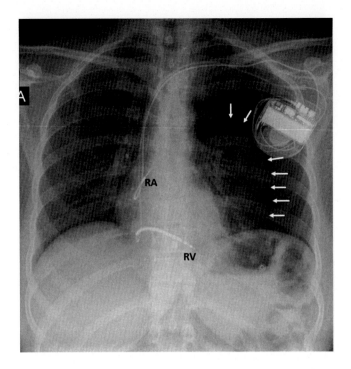

FIG. 2

Severe pneumothorax in a patient with a dual-chamber defibrillator. The right atrial (RA) lead was implanted in the right atrial appendage and the right ventricular (RV) lead at the apex. *White arrows* show the line between the collapsed left lung and the ribcage in a posteroanterior view. Note that there is no lung vasculature between this line and the ribcage.

Hemothorax is an accumulation of air and blood. In this situation, there is an air-fluid level in addition to radiographic evidence of air accumulation in the pleural space (Fig. 6).

Cardiac perforation

Atrial or ventricular leads may occasionally perforate the heart chamber [1]. Cardiac perforation may be easily detected in a PA view (Fig. 7). However, some cases may need a lateral view for a final confirmation. In the lateral view, the normally located RV lead's tip distance from the sternum is more than 3 mm. Any distance less than 3 mm, especially crossing the epicardial fat line, indicates lead penetration (Fig. 8).

Ventricular lead placement within the middle cardiac vein may mimic cardiac perforation. In this situation, the pacing threshold usually increases and the ECG shows a right bundle branch block pattern. The lateral view of CXR can easily detect this complication. In this situation, RV lead orientation is toward the posterior part of the heart (Fig. 9).

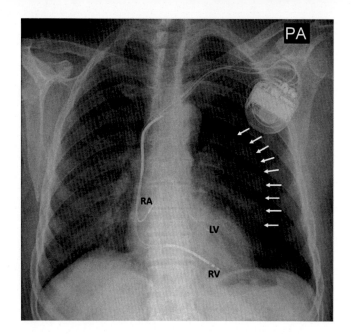

FIG. 3

Severe pneumothorax in a patient with a biventricular defibrillator (CRT–D). The right atrial (RA) lead was implanted in the right atrial appendage, the right ventricular (RV) lead at the apex, and the left ventricular (LV) lead within the lateral cardiac vein. *White arrows* show the line between the collapsed left lung and the ribcage in a posteroanterior view. Note that there is no lung vasculature between this line and the ribcage. CRT–D: cardiac resynchronization therapy defibrillator.

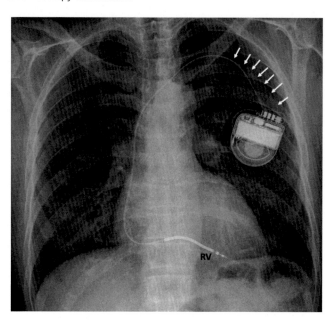

FIG. 4

Mild pneumothorax in a patient with a single-chamber defibrillator. The right ventricular (RV) lead is properly placed at the apex. *White arrows* show a barely visible pneumothorax line in the posteroanterior view. Note that the black shadow of pneumothorax is limited to the apical portion of the left lung.

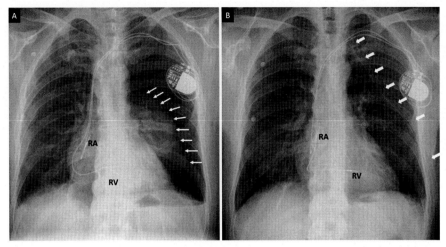

FIG. 5

Resolution of the pneumothorax after air drainage for the left pleural space using a chest tube. Right atrial (RA) and right ventricular (RV) leads are properly placed within the heart. Panel A shows a massive pneumothorax in the patient with a dual-chamber pacemaker. Note that the left lung completely collapsed and retracted to the left hilum. Lung border is shown by thin white arrows. Panel B shows complete air drainage from the left pleural space by the chest tube (*thick white arrows*).

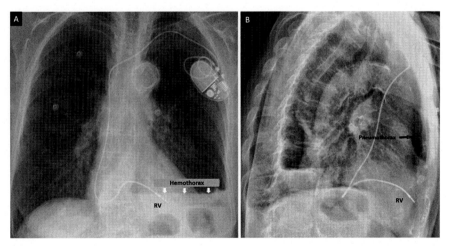

FIG. 6

Hemopneumothorax in a patient with a single-chamber pacemaker. The right ventricular (RV) lead is deeply implanted within the RV apex. Panel A clearly shows the air-fluid level (hemothorax, *white arrows*) in the posteroanterior view. Although no clear pneumothorax line is seen, a flat line is indicative of mixed air and fluid. Panel B, however, depicts air accumulation behind the sternum (pneumothorax, *black arrow*).

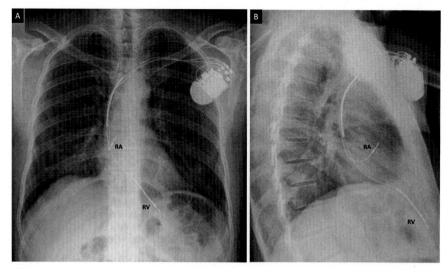

FIG. 7

Perforated right ventricular (RV) defibrillator lead in a patient with a dual-chamber defibrillator. The posteroanterior view (Panel A) shows a right atrial (RA) lead within the appendage and an RV lead tip in an unusual location beneath the left hemidiaphragm. The lateral view (Panel B) clearly shows that the RV lead tip is located outside the cardiac shadow in a space between the xiphoid process and the diaphragm.

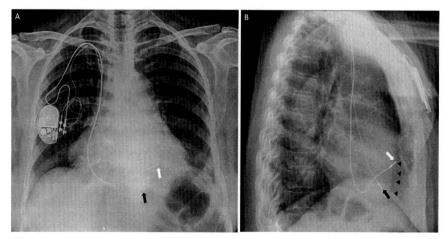

FIG. 8

Penetrated right ventricular (RV) pacing lead in a patient with a multifocal RV pacemaker. The posteroanterior view (Panel A) shows a passive lead (*black arrow*) near the RV apex and another active lead (*white arrow*) implanted in the upper septal area. Both leads are seen inside the cardiac silhouette. The lateral view (Panel B) again shows a passive lead (*black arrow*) location near the apex; however, the active lead tip (*white arrow*) is penetrated into the epicardial fat line (*black arrowheads*). This latter finding is an early sign of lead perforation.

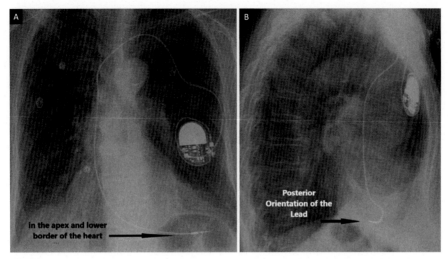

FIG. 9

Inadvertent right ventricular (RV) lead implantation within the middle cardiac vein. In the posteroanterior view (Panel A), the RV lead course is similar to the lead placement within the RV apex; however, the lateral view (Panel B) shows that the RV lead oriented posteriorly.

Loose connection

When the leads are properly connected to the generator, terminal pins extend beyond the distal connecting blocks. In case of loose connections (loose set screw), the lead pin disengages from the generator connector blocks and the terminal pins are not extended beyond the connecting blocks (Figs. 10 and 11). After lead reconnection, CXRs help us to confirm the correct lead connection (Figs. 10 and 11).

Lead dislodgements

All CIED leads may dislodge from the implantation sites [2]. Left ventricular leads are the most susceptible leads for dislodgement (Fig. 12). At present, lead dislodgement is very rare in active fixation leads. However, atrial or right ventricular leads may dislocate from the initially implanted locations (Figs. 13 and 14). Dislodgements could be macro or micro. Only macrodislodgements are detected by CXR images.

Lead fracture

Lead fracture is an important malfunction after pacemaker implantation. It usually occurs at the junction of the clavicle and the first rib (Figs. 15–17). However, fractures in the intracardiac part of CIED leads are not infrequent. Lead fractures need lead replacements.

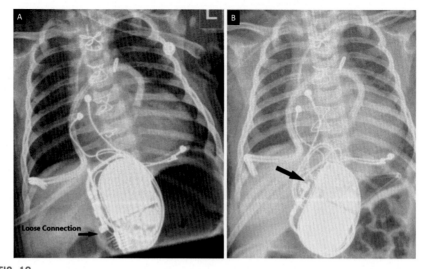

FIG. 10

Loose connection in a patient with an epicardial pacemaker. Panel A shows that the terminal pin is not extended beyond the distal connecting block (*black arrow*). Panel B shows appropriate terminal pin engagement after lead reconnection (*black arrow*).

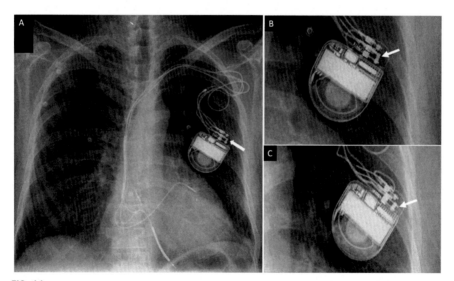

FIG. 11

Loose connection in a patient with a biventricular defibrillator. Panel A shows that the terminal pin of the right ventricular (RV) lead is not extended beyond the distal connecting block (*middle row, white arrow*). Right atrial (RA) and left ventricular (LV) leads are appropriately connected to the generator. Panel B shows a magnified view of the generator region for better demonstration of loose connection of the RV lead (*white arrow*). In a biventricular device, terminal pins of the pacing leads are connected to the generator according the predefined sequence: atrial lead to the top port, RV lead to the middle port, and LV lead to the bottom port. Panel C shows that after lead reconnection, the terminal pin of the RV lead is clearly extended beyond the distal connecting blocks (*white arrow*).

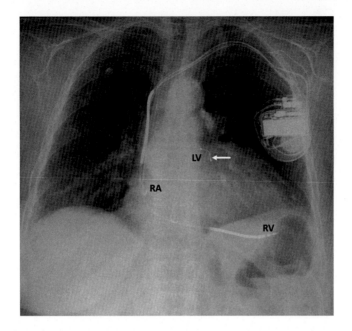

FIG. 12

Posteroanterior (PA) and lateral (LAT) chest radiographs showing a cardiac resynchronization therapy device with a dislodged left ventricular (LV) lead. Note that right atrial (RA) and right ventricular (RV) defibrillator leads are in the correct position within the RA appendage and the RV apex. The LV lead (*black arrow*) is dislocated into the coronary sinus from vein branch (*white arrow*).

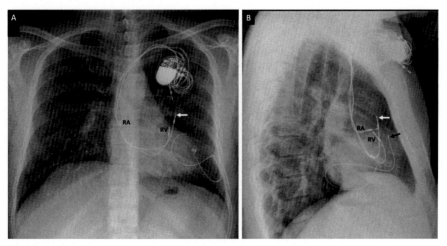

FIG. 13

Posteroanterior (PA) and lateral (LAT) chest radiographs showing a dual-chamber pacemaker with a dislodged right ventricular (RV) lead. Panel A shows the right atrial (RA) lead has lost its "J-curve" but it is still attached to the appendage. The abandoned fractured RV lead was fixed to the RV outflow tract. A new ventricular lead (*white arrow*) was seen outside the cardiac silhouette (suspicious to perforation). There is also an old cut epicardial active lead (*black arrow*). Panel B confirms that the new ventricular lead actually dislocated into the pulmonary trunk (*white arrow*) and ruled out cardiac perforation. Note that the dislodged lead is located within the cardiac silhouette and enters the pulmonary trunk through the outflow tract.

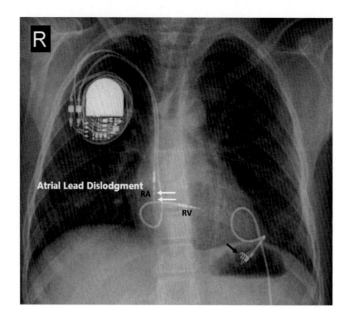

FIG. 14

Posteroanterior chest radiographs showing a dual-chamber pacemaker with right atrial (RA) lead dislodgement. Note that the RA lead lost its "J-curve" without any attachment to the atrial wall (*white arrows*). The right ventricular (RV) lead is adequately attached to the interventricular septum. There is an abandoned active epicardial lead (*black arrow*).

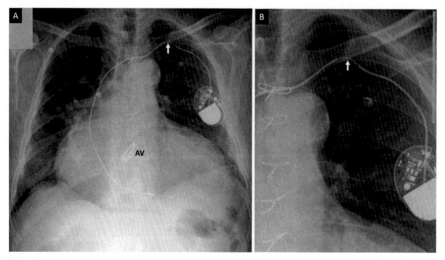

FIG. 15

Posteroanterior chest radiographs showing a single-chamber pacemaker with a right ventricular lead fracture in a patient with aortic valve (AV) prosthesis. Panel A shows the lead fracture (*white arrow*) that occurred at its typical location (junction of the clavicle and the first rib). Panel B shows a magnified image showing partial fracture involving the outer layer helix (*white arrow*).

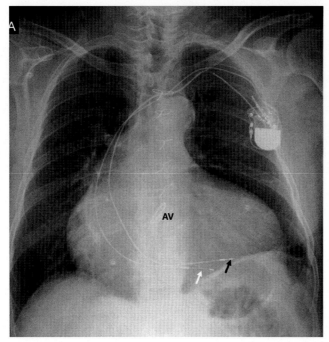

FIG. 16

Posteroanterior chest radiograph of the same patient depicted in Fig. 15 after new ventricular lead implantation. An old fractured lead is a bipolar passive lead (*white arrow*). A new lead is a bipolar active fixation lead (*black arrow*). *AV*, aortic valve prosthesis.

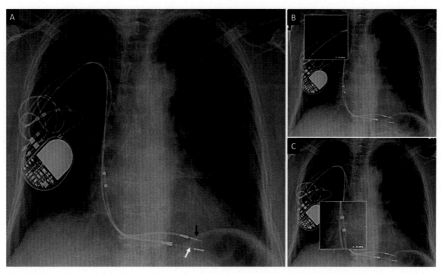

FIG. 17

Posteroanterior chest radiographs showing a single-lead atrial-sensing ventricular pacemaker (VDD pacemaker) with lead fracture. Panel A shows a dual-chamber pacemaker with two leads: a fracture VDD lead (*white arrow*) and a new active ventricular lead (*black arrow*). Panel B shows a magnified image from the first fracture site near the junction of the clavicle and the first rib. Panel C shows a magnified image at the second fracture site near the atrial-sensing electrodes.

References

[1] A.P. Vanezis, R. Prasad, R. Andrews, Pacemaker leads and cardiac perforation, JRSM Open 8 (3) (2017), https://doi.org/10.1177/2054270416681432, 2054270416681432.

[2] B. Fuertes, J. Toquero, R. Arroyo-Espliguero, I.F. Lozano, Pacemaker lead displacement: mechanisms and management, Indian Pacing Electrophysiol J 3 (4) (2003) 231–238.

Novel cardiac implantable electronic devices

6

Majid Haghjoo[a,b,*]

aDepartment of Cardiac Electrophysiology, Rajaie Cardiovascular Medical and Research Center,
Iran University of Medical Sciences, Tehran, Iran
bCardiac Electrophysiology Research Center, Rajaie Cardiovascular Medical and Research
Center, Iran University of Medical Sciences, Tehran, Iran
*Corresponding author: majid.haghjoo@gmail.com

Key Points

- Subcutaneous implantable cardioverter defibrillators, leadless pacemakers, and His pacing are important novel tools in the treatment and management of life-threatening ventricular arrhythmias and symptomatic bradyarrhythmias.

- As these devices become more commonly used in clinical practice, the physicians' understanding of these devices and their utility is paramount for patient follow-up and detection of potential complications.

Introduction

A subcutaneous implantable cardioverter defibrillator (S-ICD) is an alternative to a transvenous ICD (T-ICD) for prevention of sudden cardiac death [1]. In 2012, the Food and Drug Administration (FDA) approved the first entirely subcutaneous implantable defibrillator. While the basic components of an S-ICD are similar to that of the traditional T-ICD, i.e., a pulse generator and a defibrillator coil, there are significant differences.

A leadless pacemaker is 93% smaller than a transvenous pacemaker [2]. This device has no separate lead and is implanted directly into the right ventricle via a transvenous femoral approach. It requires no subcutaneous pocket. At present, only one leadless pacemaker (Micra TPS, Medtronic, Minneapolis, MN) has been approved by the US Food and Drug Administration for use.

His pacing is a new pacing technique to reduce ventricular dyssynchrony and provide a more physiologic pattern of activation via His–Purkinje activation [3]. His pacing is performed using a non-stylet-driven active fixation lead (69 cm Select Secure 3830 Medtronic lead).

In this chapter, we familiarize physicians and other health-care providers with these devices using chest radiography (CXR) images taken in different views.

Radiographic Atlas of Cardiac Implantable Electronic Devices. https://doi.org/10.1016/B978-0-323-84753-7.00006-6

Subcutaneous implantable cardioverter defibrillators

An S-ICD is composed of three components (Fig. 1):

- A pulse generator, implanted in the left lateral position in the midaxillary line at the level of the fifth and sixth intercostal spaces.
- Two sensing electrodes lying directly before and after a defibrillator coil.
- A parasternal defibrillator coil, implanted parallel to the left sternal border.

Chest radiographs (CXRs) are very important in evaluating the PRAETORIAN score for predicting successful defibrillation testing [4]. The score can be applied only to the S-ICD systems implanted within the anatomical area, as shown in Fig. 2. The score measurement consists of three steps (Table 1):

Step 1: Determine the number of coil widths of the fat tissue between the nearest half of the S-ICD coil and the sternum or ribs using the coil width as a reference (Figs. 3 and 4). In case of ≤ 1 coil width of the fat tissue, a score of 30 points is rewarded; the score of Step 1 increases to 60 in case of > 1 but ≤ 2 coil widths and to 90 in case of > 2 but ≤ 3 coil widths. In the first step, a maximum score of 150 points can be rewarded in case of > 3 coil widths of the fat tissue.

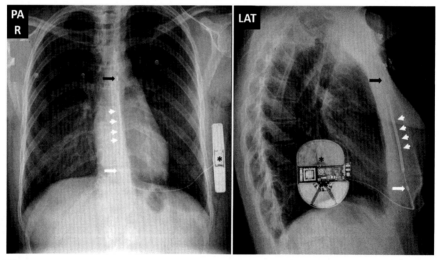

FIG. 1

Posteroanterior (PA) and lateral (LAT) chest radiographic views in a patient with a subcutaneous implantable cardiac defibrillator (SICD). SICD consists of two components: one generator is located in the axillary area (*) and a single lead tunneled subcutaneously from the axillary pocket to the left parasternal border. The SICD lead has one defibrillation coil (*white arrowheads*) that is flanked by two sensing electrodes, namely, the proximal-sensing electrode (*white arrow*) before coil and the distal-sensing electrode (*black arrow*) after coil.

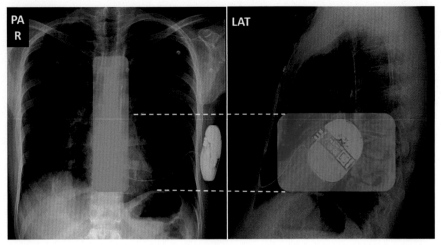

FIG. 2

Minimum requirements in chest radiography for determining the PRAETORIAN score. The coil should be in the green-shaded area of the PA view, and the cranial side of the generator has to project over the lateral portion of the heart in the *green-shaded area* of the LAT view and between the *white dash line* in the PA view.

Table 1 Steps for PRAETORIAN score determination using posteroanterior and lateral chest radiographs.

Step	Description
Step 1	Determine the number of coil widths of fat between the nearest half of the ICD coil and the sternum or ribs: – score 30 for ≤1 coil width – score 60 for >1 but ≤2 coil widths – score 90 for >2 but ≤3 coil widths – score 150 for >3 coil widths
Step 2	Determine the position of the S-ICD generator in relation to the midline: – step 1 score × 1 if the generator is on or posterior to this line – step 1 score × 2 if the entire generator is anterior to this line – step 1 score × 4 if the posterior side of the generator is >4 cm anterior to this line
Step 3	Determine the amount of fat between the generator and the thoracic wall: – step 2 score × 1 if amount of fat is <1 generator width – step 2 score × 1.5 if amount of fat is >1 generator width
Step 4	Body mass index (BMI) correction: – BMI ≤25 kg/m^2, final score minus 40 – BMI >25 kg/m^2, no change is needed

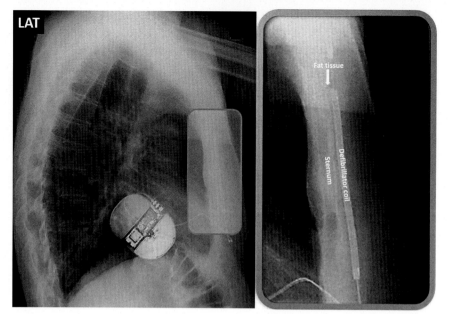

FIG. 3

Example of small subcoil fat in the lateral (LAT) chest radiographic view. Note that there is less than one coil width of fat tissue between the nearest half of the shock coil and the sternum. Therefore, the Step 1 score in this example is 30 points.

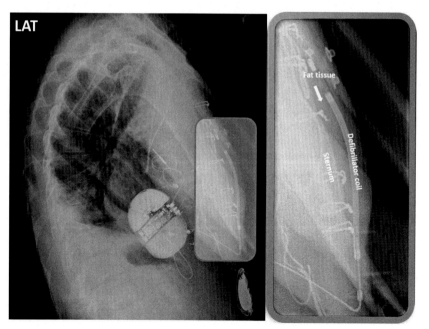

FIG. 4

Example of moderate subcoil fat in the lateral (LAT) chest radiographic view. Note that there are at least two coil widths of fat tissue between the nearest half of the shock coil and the sternum. Therefore, the Step 1 score in this example is 60.

Step 2: Determine the position of the S-ICD generator in relation to the midline (Figs. 5 and 6): In order to accurately determine the generator position, first the ventral and dorsal lung borders are defined. Then, a perpendicular line from the sternum through the generator to the dorsal lung border is drawn. After that, the S-ICD generator position is determined relative to the middle of this line. When the generator is positioned on or posterior to the middle line, the S-ICD generator is in an optimal position and the Step 1 score is then multiplied by 1. When the entire generator is positioned anterior to this line, the score is multiplied by 2. In extreme cases in which the posterior side of the generator is positioned more than half a generator length (i.e., 4 cm) anterior to the middle line, the score is multiplied by 4.

Step 3: Determine the amount of the fat tissue between the nearest point of the generator and the thoracic wall using the width of the generator as reference (Fig. 7). When < 1 generator width of fat is visualized between the nearest point of the generator and the chest wall, then the Step 2 score is multiplied by 1. When > 1 generator width of the fat tissue is detected between the generator and the chest wall, then the Step 2 score is multiplied by 1.5.

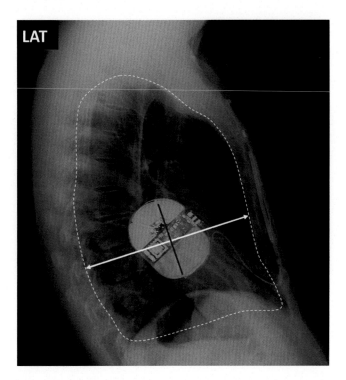

FIG. 5

Example of optimal generator position in the lateral (LAT) chest radiographic view. Note that the generator is on the *red line* (middle of the perpendicular line drawn from the sternum to the dorsal lung border), the S-ICD generator is in optimal position, and the Step 1 score is multiplied by 1.

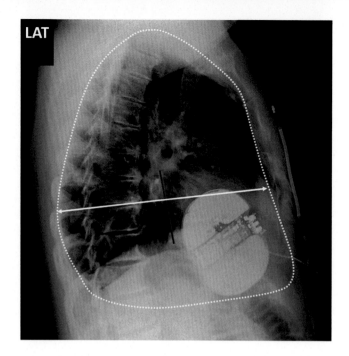

FIG. 6

Example of nonoptimal generator position in the lateral (LAT) chest radiographic view. Note that the entire generator is positioned anterior to the *red line*; therefore, the Step 1 score is multiplied by 2.

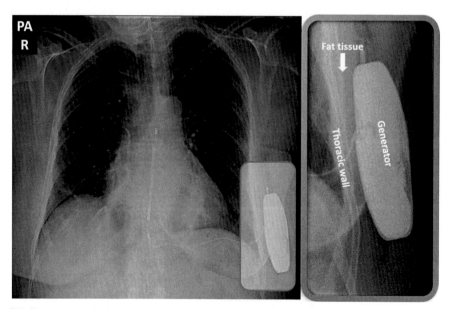

FIG. 7

Example of optimal subgenerator fat tissue in the posteroanterior (PA) chest radiographic view. Note that there is less than one generator width of fat between the nearest point of the generator and the chest wall; therefore, the Step 2 score is multiplied by 1.

Body mass index (BMI) correction: In case of the PRAETORIAN score ≥ 90, patients with a BMI $\leq 25\,kg/m^2$ are rewarded by subtracting 40 points. In those with BMI $> 25\,kg/m^2$, the score remained unchanged.

DFT success is predicted by the final PRAETORIAN score:

1. PRAETORIAN score < 90 points: low risk for conversion failure of ventricular arrhythmias.
2. PRAETORIAN score ≥ 90 and < 150 points: a first shock efficacy of $< 90\%$ is expected for this group, but they will still be able to convert with repetitive shocks.
3. PRAETORIAN score of ≥ 150: high risk for conversion failure of ventricular arrhythmias even with repetitive shocks.

Combined SICDs and conventional pacemakers

At present, SICDs do not provide adequate pacing support. Therefore, it is not unusual to see a combination of SICDs and epicardial pacemakers (Fig. 8).

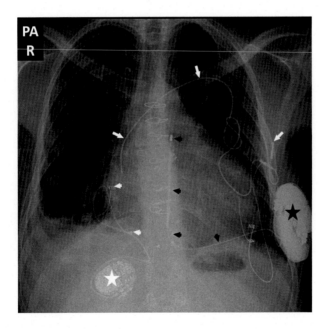

FIG. 8

Combined subcutaneous implantable cardiac defibrillator (SICD) and conventional pacemaker. In this patient with a history of prior endocardial pacemaker infection (remnants of the lead is shown in *white arrows*), an epicardial pacemaker (*white star* and *arrowheads*) is implanted. Then, an SICD (*black star* and *arrowheads*) was implanted because of ventricular fibrillation during hospitalization.

Leadless pacemaker

This pacemaker is attached via 4 Nitinol FlexFix tines into the right ventricle (RV) myocardium. On CXR, an RV leadless pacemaker appears as a linear radiopaque device implanted into the right ventricular wall (Figs. 9 and 10). Potential complications include device dislodgement, cardiac perforation, elevated pacing thresholds requiring device retrieval and reimplantation, and vascular complications. Dislodgement and cardiac perforation can be identified on CXRs.

His pacing

His bundle pacing is a relatively novel method of cardiac pacing. This method is used in patients with an atrioventricular block to help prevent right ventricular pacing-induced heart failure and in patients with a bundle branch block and cardiomyopathy to normalize electrical conduction through the His–Purkinje system. A His pacing lead is implanted in the mid-septum very close to the tricuspid annulus on CXR (Figs. 11 and 12).

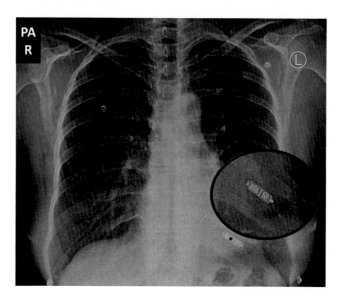

FIG. 9

Posteroanterior (PA) chest radiographic view in a patient with a Micra leadless pacemaker. Note that the Micra pacemaker (*black star*) is implanted in the apicoseptal area. The Micra implantation area is magnified for better illustration.

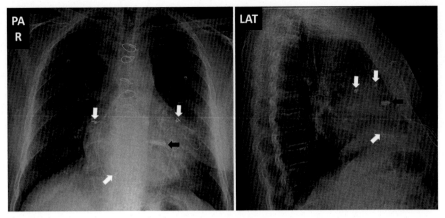

FIG. 10

Posteroanterior (PA) and lateral (LAT) chest radiographic views in a patient with a Micra leadless pacemaker. Note that the Micra pacemaker is implanted in the mid-septal area (*black arrow*). Prior epicardial pacemaker leads are shown by *white arrows*.

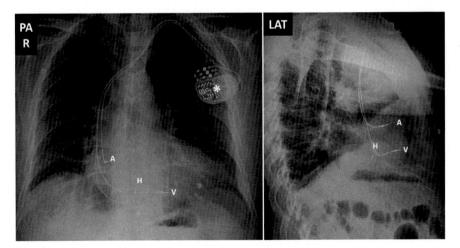

FIG. 11

Posteroanterior (PA) and lateral (LAT) chest radiographic views of His pacing in a patient with a triple-chamber pacemaker (*white star*). Note that the atrial lead is implanted in the right atrial appendage (A), the right ventricular lead (V) in the low septal area, and the His pacing lead (H) in the His recording area near the superior portion of the tricuspid annulus.

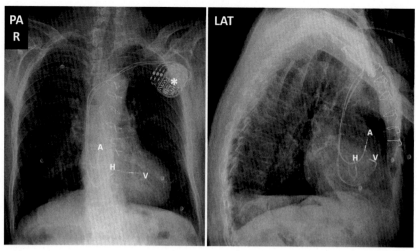

FIG. 12

Posteroanterior (PA) and lateral (LAT) chest radiographic views of His pacing in a patient with a triple-chamber pacemaker (*white star*). Note that the atrial lead is implanted in the right atrial appendage (A), the right ventricular lead (V) in the high septal area, and His pacing lead (H) in the His recording area near the superior portion of the tricuspid annulus.

References

[1] M.C. Burke, M.R. Gold, B.P. Knight, C.S. Barr, D.A.M.J. Theuns, L.V.A. Boersma, R.E. Knops, R. Weiss, A.R. Leon, J.M. Herre, M. Husby, K.M. Stein, P.D. Lambiase, Safety and efficacy of the totally subcutaneous implantable defibrillator: 2-year results from a pooled analysis of the IDE study and EFFORTLESS registry, J Am Coll Cardiol 65 (16) (2015) 1605–1615, https://doi.org/10.1016/j.jacc.2015.02.047. 25908064.

[2] D. Reynolds, G.Z. Duray, R. Omar, K. Soejima, P. Neuzil, S. Zhang, C. Narasimhan, C. Steinwender, J. Brugada, M. Lloyd, P.R. Roberts, V. Sagi, J. Hummel, M.G. Bongiorni, R.E. Knops, C.R. Ellis, C.C. Gornick, M.A. Bernabei, V. Laager, K. Stromberg, E.R. Williams, J.H. Hudnall, P. Ritter, Micra Transcatheter Pacing Study Group, A leadless intracardiac transcatheter pacing system, New Engl J Med 374 (6) (2016) 533–541, https://doi.org/10.1056/NEJMoa1511643. Epub 2015 Nov 9 26551877.

[3] A.J.M. Lewis, P. Foley, Z. Whinnett, D. Keene, B. Chandrasekaran, His bundle pacing: a new strategy for physiological ventricular activation, J Am Heart Assoc 8 (6) (2019), https://doi.org/10.1161/JAHA.118.010972, e010972. Erratum in: J Am Heart Assoc. 2019 Jun 4;8(11):e002310.

[4] A.B.E. Quast, S.W.E. Baalman, T.F. Brouwer, L. Smeding, A.A.M. Wilde, M.C. Burke, R.E. Knops, A novel tool to evaluate the implant position and predict defibrillation success of the subcutaneous implantable cardioverter-defibrillator: the PRAETORIAN score, Heart Rhythm 16 (3) (2019) 403–410, https://doi.org/10.1016/j.hrthm.2018.09.029. Epub 2018 Oct 4 30292861.

Implantable cardiac monitors

7

Farzad Kamali[a,b,*]

[a]Department of Cardiac Electrophysiology, Rajaie Cardiovascular Medical and Research Center,
Iran University of Medical Sciences, Tehran, Iran
[b]Cardiac Electrophysiology Research Center, Rajaie Cardiovascular Medical and Research
Center, Iran University of Medical Sciences, Tehran, Iran
*Corresponding author: kamali.farzad@gmail.com

Key Points

- An implantable cardiac monitor (ICM) is a small device inserted subcutaneously for continuous electrocardiogram monitoring.
- This device is detectable with chest radiography. Therefore, a correct identification of this device is very crucial to all physicians.

Introduction

An implantable cardiac monitor (ICM) is a small device inserted subcutaneously for continuous cardiac electrocardiogram monitoring [1]. The battery longevity of ICMs is about 3–4 years. ICM has a loop memory that continually analyzes and records the ECG. Arrhythmic events are recorded and memorized automatically on the basis of a predefined algorithm or by patients when they experience symptoms. In this chapter, we discuss the radiographic presentations of different kinds of currently available ICMs.

Indications for ICM

ICMs are most commonly utilized in the evaluation of selected patients with unexplained syncope and palpitation as well as for the detection of subclinical AF.

Optimal position for ICM

Subcutaneous implantation of an ICM requires a minor invasive procedure. The electrocardiogram is measured between the two ends of the device. Therefore, the best

Radiographic Atlas of Cardiac Implantable Electronic Devices. https://doi.org/10.1016/B978-0-323-84753-7.00007-8

position for an ICM is 45 degrees to the sternum over the left fourth intercostal space, although its implantation parallel to the sternum is also accepted. Optimal ICM positioning is associated with a larger "QRS" or "R" wave amplitude (ideally $\geq 0.3\,\text{mV}$ on the programmer), better detection of "P" and "R" waves, and reduction of P or T wave oversensing (Figs. 1–4).

The most common ICM models are manufactured by Medtronic [2] (Reveal XT and Reveal LINQ), Abott [3] (Confirm and Confirm Rx), and Biotronic [4] (BioMonitor 2 and BioMonitor 3). Most of the ICMs such as the Reveal LINQ and BioMonitors are MRI conditional. Earlier devices needed a small surgical incision for implantation, while recent, smaller models such as the Reveal LINQ (Fig. 5), Confirm Rx, and BioMonitor 3 are easily implanted by subcutaneous injection via an incision smaller than 1 cm.

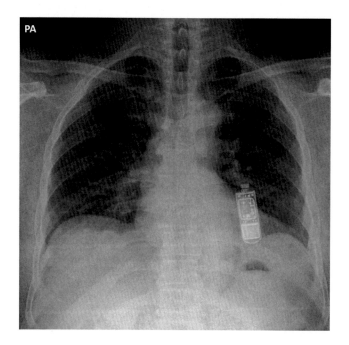

FIG. 1

Posteroanterior (PA) chest radiograph of a patient with an ICM (Medtronic Reveal XT). On a CXR, the ICM appears like a USB flash drive without wires attached to it. The position and angle of the ICM in this patient is appropriate.

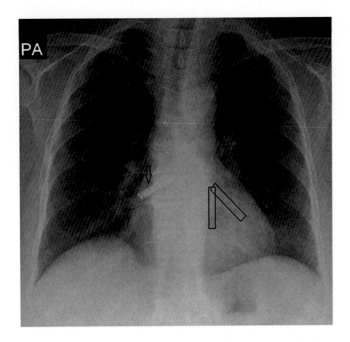

FIG. 2

Posteroanterior chest radiograph (PA) showing an ICM (Medtronic LINQ) in an inappropriate position (*black arrow*). The appropriate positions for ICMs show on the chest radiograph, schematically.

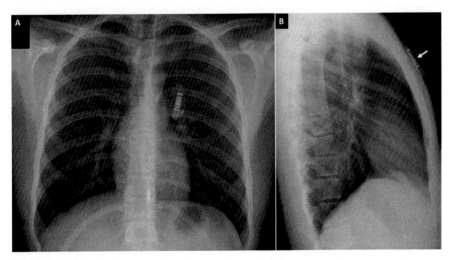

FIG. 3

Posteroanterior (A) and lateral (B) views of chest radiographs showing an ICM (Medtronic LINQ) over the left anterior chest wall. Note that the ICM is shown by a *small white arrow* on the lateral view.

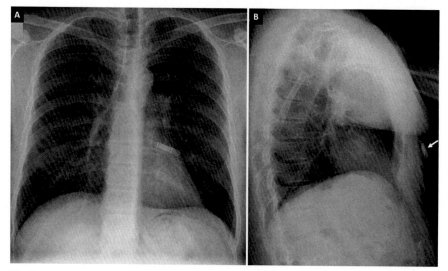

FIG. 4

Posteroanterior (A) and lateral (B) views of chest radiographs of an ICM implanted lower than the preferred site (left fourth intercostal space). The ICM is depicted by a small *white arrow* on the lateral view.

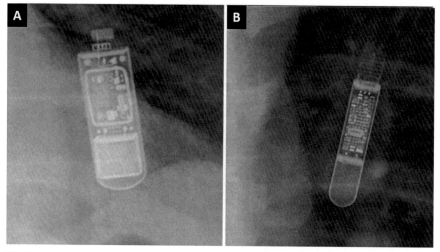

FIG. 5

Magnified views of the common types of ICMs in the market. (A) Medtronic Reveal XT: the size is larger compared with Reveal LINQ. (B) Medtronic Reveal LINQ: smaller device with easier implantation.

References

[1] S. Giancaterino, F. Lupercio, M. Nishimura, J.C. Hsu, Current and future use of insertable cardiac monitors, JACC Clin Electrophysiol 4 (11) (2018) 1383–1396.

[2] Medtronic, Reveal LINQ Insertable Cardiac Monitoring System. http://www.medtronicdiagnostics.com/us/cardiac-monitors/reveal-linq/index.htm. (Accessed June 2021).

[3] St. Jude Medical/Abbott, Implantable Cardiac Monitors. https://www.cardiovascular.abbott/us/en/hcp/products/cardiac-rhythm-management/insertable-cardiac-monitors/confirm-rx.html. (Accessed June 2021).

[4] Biotronik, BioMonitor III. Available at. https://www.biotronik.com/en-us/products/crm/arrhythmia-monitoring/biomonitor-3. (Accessed June 2021).

Index

Note: Page numbers followed by *f* indicate figures and *t* indicate tables.